Table of Contents

How to Use the Trainer's Guide

The guide is divided into four sections:
I.   Adult Learning Principles
II. Plan
III. Implement
IV. Summary and Conclusion

Appendix B contains worksheets and tools to help you apply the information to future trainings. You may choose to read this guide from cover to cover and then apply the information to a training or you may want to use sections or tools as a reference during planning or implementation of your training session. The following table provides an overview of each section and its contents.

Trainer's Guide Overview

I. Adult Learning Principles	1. Introduction 2. Principles of adult learning (underscores the importance of using the adult learning cycle to help participants apply skills learned beyond the training) 3. Assess participants' strengths and needs to design an appropriate training
II. Plan	1. Defining an appropriate plan, training goals, and objectives 2. Selecting appropriate training methods (seven commonly used training methods are explained) 3. Principles for selecting and using audiovisual materials 4. Tips for developing a realistic, responsive training plan
III. Implement	1. Ways to create a safe and comfortable learning environment 2. Tips on facilitating the training, including giving feedback, managing time, and ensuring cultural sensitivity 3. Ways to actively engage participants using icebreakers and energizers 4. Ideas on how to provide closure 5. Evaluation methods
IV. Summary and Conclusion	Puts it all together
Appendixes	Appendix A provides examples of icebreakers, energizers, closing activities, and training evaluations Appendix B contains worksheets to apply concepts and tips discussed throughout the guide

I. Adult Learning Principles

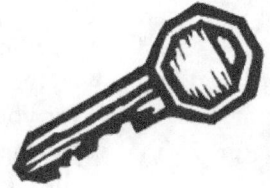

1. Introduction

Education is one tool in the fight against cancer. Fully informed health care professionals and consumers can act more effectively to care for their patients, themselves, and their loved ones. It is vitally important that everyone learn how to decrease their risks for getting cancer, the importance of screening and early detection, and ways to access various treatment options.

Cancer education can take many forms: individual counseling and education, group training sessions, media campaigns, and printed materials such as brochures, pamphlets, and newsletters. This trainer's guide is designed for both lay people and health professionals who are conducting group-training sessions with community and scientific audiences. It offers practical suggestions for taking your knowledge, tailoring it to the specific needs of your audience, and packaging the information in new ways. The guide provides ways to enliven your training, encourage more active participation, and enrich the learning experience for everyone involved.

The trainer's guide also provides examples of icebreakers, energizers, and closing activities as well as checklists and charts to help you write objectives, develop a training plan, and conduct an evaluation.

Guiding principles that serve as underpinnings for the development of this trainer's guide are:

- *We all have incredible assets to bring to the training experience.* You, as trainers, already have a wealth of information and skills. This trainer's guide is merely an opportunity to review, refresh, and reinvigorate your training. This guide also describes ways to elicit the experiences and skills of your participants so that they are actively engaged in the learning experience.

• *Application is an important part of any learning experience.* Just as the trainer's guide encourages you to construct opportunities for your participants to apply their new information and skills during your training, it also provides you with a chance to do the same. Most sections have worksheets that give you an opportunity to apply the information from that section.

• *Changes in knowledge, attitudes and behaviors, and skills are primary objectives.* The trainer's guide provides suggestions for ways to use training methods that lead to increased information and skill acquisition, and to improved attitudes.

2. Principles of Adult Learning

All trainers should understand the principles of adult learning; however, cancer education poses some unique challenges. The word "cancer" still strikes fear in the hearts and minds of many people. Participants in your training sessions may come with a number of emotions, unresolved feelings, fears, and concerns that will influence their receptivity to the training content. They also may bring experiences, perspectives, and insights that will enrich the training. Thus, cancer education is not just a matter of presenting new information to a passive, receptive audience. The trainer must carefully consider the emotional context in which this education takes place.

Malcolm Knowles, often referred to as the "father of adult education," found that adult learning occurs best when it follows certain principles. If trainers follow these guidelines, they will greatly enhance the learning experience for participants (Knowles, 1990). Arnold et al. (1991), among other adult educators, state that people retain:

- 20 percent of what they **hear**
- 30 percent of what they **see**
- 50 percent of what they **see** and **hear**
- 70 percent of what they **see, hear,** and **say** (e.g. discuss, explain to others)
- 90 percent of what they **see, hear, say**, and **do**

EXAMPLE

Therefore, for participants to retain what they learn in cancer education workshops, they need a chance not only to **hear** a lecture or discussion, **see** a demonstration or visual aids, and discuss the material, but they must also have an opportunity to **do** something with the new information and skills. This can take the form of applying their new insights to a case study or role play exercise, or it can take the form of developing an action plan of ways to use their training insights in real life.

It is also important to remember the adult learning cycle. Participatory training is the hallmark of adult learning. It moves participants through the four phases of the adult learning cycle described on page 7.

Participants learn best when...	The role of the trainer is to...
• They feel valued and respected for the experiences and perspectives they bring to the training situation	• Elicit participants' experiences and perspectives
• The learning experience is active and not passive	• Actively engage participants in their learning experience
• The learning experience actually fills their immediate needs	• Identify participants' needs and tie training concepts into these identified needs
• They accept responsibility for their own learning	• Make sure that training content and skills are directly relevant to participants' experiences so that they will want to learn
• Their learning is self-directed and meaningful to them	• Involve participants in deciding on the content and skills that will be covered during the training
• Their learning experience addresses ideas, feelings, and actions	• Use multiple training methods that address knowledge, attitudes, and skills
• New material is related to what participants already know	• Use training methods that enable participants to establish this relationship and integration of new material
• The learning environment is conducive to learning	• Take measures to ensure that the physical and social environment (training space) is safe, comfortable, and enjoyable
• Learning is reinforced	• Use training methods that allow participants to practice new skills and ensure prompt, reinforcing feedback
• Learning is applied immediately	• Provide opportunities for participants to apply the new information and skills they have learned
• Learning occurs in small groups	• Use training methods that encourage participants to explore feelings, attitudes, and skills with other learners
• The trainer values their contributions as both a learner and a teacher	• Encourage participants to share their expertise and experiences with others

Using the Adult Learning Cycle

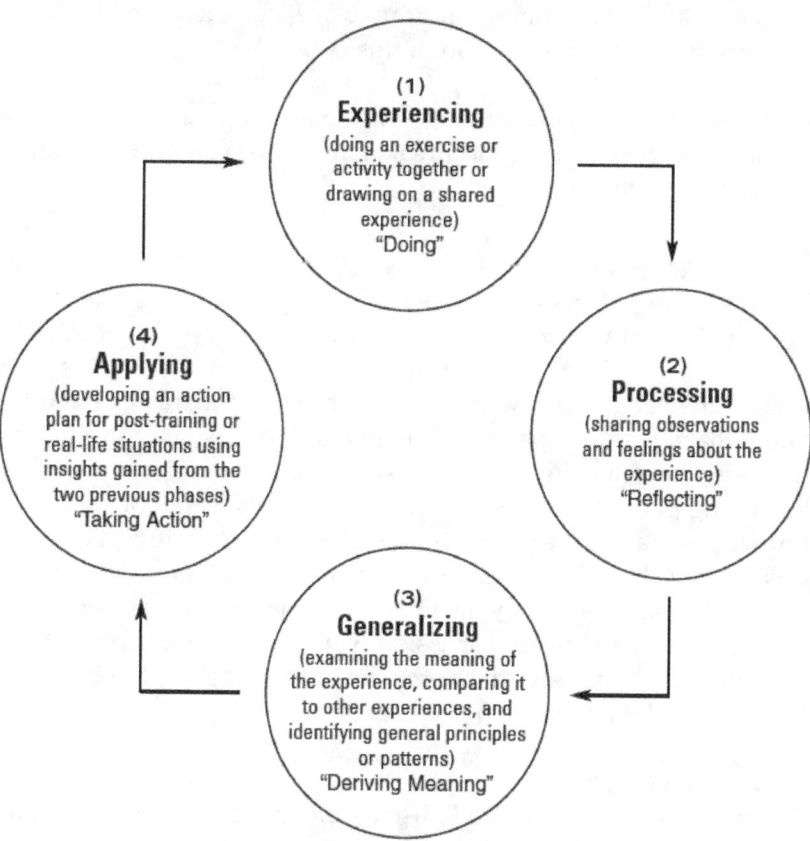

It is important to move participants through this cycle at least once per module or 4-hour session. If your training will be more than 4 hours in length, it will be necessary to complete proportionately more full cycles.

Applying the Adult Learning Cycle to Cancer Education: An Example

Let's look at how a training program on cancer survivorship might move participants through this cycle.

Once the trainer has set the stage for the training, reviewed the agenda, and conducted an icebreaker, he or she can move through the adult learning cycle.

Phase 1: Experiencing

The trainer might first lead an activity designed to get participants talking about how receiving a cancer diagnosis impacts their life.

If all of the participants were cancer survivors, the trainer would know that everyone has had the experience of first learning their diagnosis, so a small group discussion might be an appropriate beginning place. However, if some participants were not survivors but were social workers from an oncology unit, the design of this activity should be modified. Since they have not necessarily personally experienced the feelings associated with a cancer diagnosis, a small group discussion would not be appropriate as a beginning place. A more appropriate beginning might be a panel presentation by a group of survivors.

Phase 2: Processing

The trainer would then lead a discussion about what people heard during their small group discussions or what feelings the panel aroused in them.

Phase 3: Generalizing

The next part of the discussion might lead to a comparison between getting a cancer diagnosis and other life-altering news.

Phase 4: Applying

The trainer would then encourage all participants to think of ways they might use these new insights. For oncology social workers, the discussion might yield insights that would help them be more compassionate and understanding with their newly-diagnosed patients. For cancer survivors, the discussion may have generated ideas to take back to their support groups or about how to get more support for themselves.

Repeating the Cycle

The trainer would then move to the next activity and the adult learning cycle would be repeated using the same structure of experiencing, processing, generalizing, and applying.

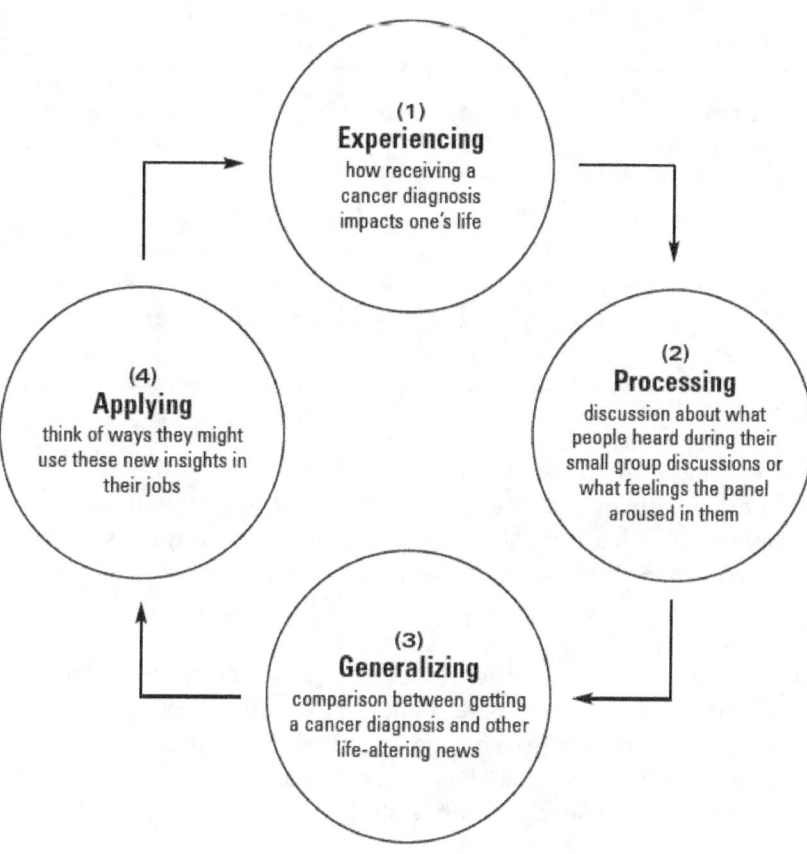

Ensuring that the Training Addresses the Fact that People Learn in Different Ways

Trainers must be aware that in any audience the participants will learn in different ways:

For participants who...	Use
• Resonate with abstract concepts and lectures	• Case studies and discussions about theories and research
• Learn best while observing others	• Demonstrations and videos
• Learn best from exercises	• Role playing and other experiential activites
• Learn best through visual means	• Videos, images, and slides

Since trainers are unlikely to know the individual learning styles of the participants in their audience, it is best to assume that there are people with all learning styles in each group and design a variety of strategies to meet the learning needs of all participants. These training methodologies will be discussed in detail in section II.2.

It is also important to consider the learning strategies to which different audiences are accustomed. For example, health care professionals are used to learning from lectures, demonstrations, and case studies. They may be less used to learning via experiential exercises and some of the creative strategies listed in section II.2. On the other hand, community members and groups of survivors or patients and family groups may prefer more interactive methods over lectures and PowerPoint presentations.

Trainers need to be judicious about matching training methodologies to the specific audience. This does *not* mean that health care professionals will never respond to experiential exercises, nor that community groups will *never* benefit from lectures. However, it does mean that training methods that the audience is not accustomed to should be used in moderation and with sensitivity.

For example, the trainer might warm up an audience of health care professionals by using experiential methods such as small group discussions about a case study *before* using role plays. Likewise, community groups might prefer lecturettes (i.e., brief lectures of no more than 15-20 minutes) followed by a question and answer period rather than a lengthy lecture.

Trainers will be most effective if they carefully consider the "culture" of their audience when choosing appropriate methodologies. In this way, participants can be carefully encouraged to explore new ways of learning.

Assisting Participants in Being Comfortable with the Learning Process

One of the trainer's primary tasks is to help participants feel comfortable with the learning process. There are many factors that hinder learning, such as fear of finding out that one's lifestyle predisposes one to a higher risk of cancer, fear of exposing one's ignorance to others, or fear of stirring up painful memories of loved ones lost to cancer. By creating a positive and non-threatening learning environment, the trainer can reassure the participants that these feelings are normal and will be carefully considered throughout the course of the training session.

3. Conducting a Participant Strengths and Needs Assessment

Before designing a program that is "one size fits all," it is important to conduct an assessment of participants' prior knowledge and experience as well as their hopes and expectations for the training. This can be accomplished through a variety of mechanisms that are employed before or at the very beginning of the training. It is important to keep in mind that training participants will bring a number of strengths and experiences as well as the need for new information, insights, and skills. Often assessments focus on "needs" but a comprehensive assessment should include both the strengths and needs of participants.

Before the Training

If you know the backgrounds of the people (i.e., general community members, health care professionals, or cancer patients and survivors) who will be participating in the training, you can conduct an assessment before planning the content and format. The best case scenario is to do this assessment with some or all of the people who will actually be participating in the training.

If you do not have a roster of who will be participating or your time is limited, another option is to conduct an assessment with key informants (i.e., people who may be demographically matched to those who will be participating, such as oncology nurses, survivors from a local support group, etc.). With this information, you will be able to design a training that builds on the strengths of the participants in order to add new information, develop new skills, and enhance understanding. Assessment methods that work well with particular participant groups include the following:

Audience	Assessment method
Health care professionals	E-mail, fax-back, or telephone surveys
Community members or survivors	Focus groups, in-person interviews, or telephone surveys

It is important to include enough people in your assessment to cover a variety of perspectives and experiences. For example, if you were conducting a community training on the importance of colorectal screening, it would be important to include a variety of health care providers (e.g., physicians, nurses, social workers, and health educators), general community members, colon cancer survivors and their family members, etc. This would give you a fuller picture of the knowledge and experience the community participants will bring to the training.

Possible questions include:
- What do participants already know about the topic?
- What experiences or insights related to the topic do participants already possess?
- What do participants believe are the challenges or barriers related to the issue? (For example, why do they think people do not avail themselves of colorectal screening services?)
- What do participants hope to gain from the training? (This includes new knowledge, skills, resources, etc.)
- What do participants desire regarding the logistics of the training (e.g., location of training, length of program, optimal number of days of training, best day of week, time of day, etc.)?

The more specific the questions, the more useful the feedback will be. You can then use the information to develop the content and format of the training as well as to guide decisions related to training logistics. Assessments can pique community members' interest in the training topic as well as gather data for planning.

If you do not have access to community members or enough time to conduct an assessment, it is also helpful to review evaluations from prior training programs.

Consider using the "Training Assessment Worksheet," in appendix B to design your own training assessment.

At the Beginning of the Training

If you are not able to conduct an assessment before the training, there are a variety of techniques that can be used to determine participants' knowledge and expertise as well as their hopes for the training that day.

Hopes and Expectations

One quick way to conduct an assessment is to ask participants to write down their hopes and expectations about the training as they arrive. One way to accomplish this assessment follows:

- Post sheets of flipchart paper on the walls of the training room with titles such as "one to two things I hope to learn at this training" and "one to two concerns I have about this training."
- Ask each participant (as they enter the training room) to write their comments on the flipchart paper.
- Review all of the comments.
- Let participants know which expectations will likely be met through the training and which may be beyond the scope of the training.

EXAMPLE

For example, if one of the participants wrote that he was concerned that the trainer would use too much technical language or difficult scientific concepts, the trainer can reassure him by saying, *"Some people seem concerned that this training will have too many concepts that are difficult to understand. We are really going to try hard to make the concepts as user-friendly as possible. However, if we start using scientific jargon or talk about things you don't understand, please let us know at that time or talk with one of the trainers during a break. We really want this training to be meaningful for everyone, so please help us by asking questions and giving us feedback."*

EXAMPLE

For another example, if someone wrote that she wanted to find specific clinical trials for a particular stage of colon cancer, the trainer might state, *"Actually, we won't be covering that specific information but I can refer you to the NCI Web site for clinical trials and give you the toll-free telephone number to call for more information."* In this manner the trainer can be a helpful resource for topics outside the scope of the training. However, if a number of participants have hopes and expectations that are not covered in your training plan, it would be helpful to take time to address these expectations **before** moving on with the training as you have planned.

This approach is respectful of peoples' perceived needs and eliminates one impediment to learning. If you feel that it is necessary, you can even revise your agenda by spending time addressing the needs of your participants and discarding a less important portion of the training. **In this case, flexibility is key.**

Group Snapshots

Another quick way to assess participants' knowledge or experience is to take a group "snapshot." To do this, give participants a series of questions, and ask for a show of hands if the question pertains to them. For example, you might ask:

- How many of you know someone who has been screened for colorectal cancer?
- How many of you know someone who has been diagnosed with colorectal cancer?
- How many of you know the screening recommendations for colorectal cancer?

This information can help the trainer structure or restructure activities to more closely draw on the participants' experiences and meet their needs.

Throughout the Training

The following strategy is not considered an assessment strategy. However, it is a way to continue the assessment process throughout the training. A good trainer is able to read the body language of the participants to ascertain the appropriateness of the content, the pace of the training, and the energy level in the group. This technique is further discussed in section III.1.

In summary, the needs and strengths assessment provides invaluable information that will assist the trainer in developing appropriate training goals and objectives.

II. Plan

1. Defining an Appropriate Plan, Training Goals, and Objectives

To develop an effective training plan that achieves the point of the educational session: i.e., to make changes in knowledge, attitudes, behaviors, and skills, a number of key questions must be answered. Some of these questions will be addressed in the needs assessment. The answers to these questions will affect the content, format, and logistics of the training. The following questions are a guide.

Questions

Who are your participants?
- What is their educational level?
- What is their experience and skill level?
- What gender and age are they?
- Are they employed?
- What kind of work do they do?
- Do they work together?
- What is their literacy level?
- How many will there be? (approximately)

When will you conduct the training?
- What day of the week?
- What time of day?
- What time of the year?
- How long will the session be?
- What will be the length of the entire program?
- How much time is there for recruitment?

Where will you conduct the training?
- What is needed?
  - What size room is needed?
  - What equipment is available?
  - What other supplies are needed?

- Location
  - Is the location accessible?
  - Is the location easy to find?
  - Can it be reached by public transportation?
  - Is there safe parking?
  - Is it handicap accessible?
  - Is it a place that does not have negative connotations for intended participants (e.g., some places are associated with poor service or indigent care, which may make some participants uncomfortable)?

What will the training involve?
- What will be the content of the training plan?
- What training tools will be needed?
- What participant materials and resources will be needed?
- Will there be advance work for participants?

What is the purpose of the training?
- What changes in knowledge, attitudes, behaviors, and skills are you hoping to accomplish through the training?
- What are the goals and objectives of the training?

How will you do it?
- How will you enroll people for the training? Some possible recruitment strategies include: flyers; PSAs on TV and radio; ads in newspapers and newsletters; and word of mouth.
- How will you engage participants?
- How will you get feedback or evaluate the effectiveness of your training?

Once these questions have been answered, the training goals and objectives can be developed. The following section provides definitions and examples of goals and objectives.

Consider using the "Questions to Help Define Appropriate Training Plan, Goals, and Objectives Worksheet" in appendix B.

Setting Goals and Objectives

Goals

Goals are broad, general statements of what one hopes to accomplish as a result of the training. An example of a goal might be:

> "Increased awareness of the importance of cancer clinical trials."

Objectives

Objectives should describe the hoped-for changes in knowledge, attitudes, skills, or behaviors in very precise terms. Usually they are written in the following manner:

> *"By the end of this training (session), participants will be able to _____."*

The word that follows 'to' should be an action <u>verb</u>.

For objectives to be helpful in determining training effectiveness, they should be measurable (e.g., *"list five common myths about mammography"* or *"compare three ways that barriers to cervical and breast cancer screening are similar"*). Attainment of training goals and objectives is one important aspect of the evaluation. Not all objectives are easily measured but most can be evaluated using standard evaluation tools or other creative strategies.

There are seven types of objectives:
• Fact
• Understanding/comprehension
• Application
• Analysis
• Synthesis
• Attitudinal
• Skill

Depending on what you hope to accomplish through the training, some or all of these types of objectives need to be developed.

Keep in mind the adult learning cycle described in section I.2 when developing your training objectives. Fact, understanding, attitudinal, and skill objectives might pertain to the *"experiencing"* part of the cycle; analysis and synthesis might pertain to the "*processing*" and "*generalizing*" parts of the cycle; and application objectives might pertain to the "*applying*" stage. Remember to move participants around the adult learning cycle at least one time per module and design objectives accordingly.

When writing the seven different types of objectives, the trainer might find the following chart of verbs helpful.

Seven Training Objective Types

1. Fact objectives:	• Define • Name • Record	• List • Repeat • State	• Recall • Recognize • Record
2. Understanding or comprehension objectives:	• Discuss • Describe • Explain	• Identify • Translate • Restate	• Express • Convert • Estimate
3. Application objectives:	• Compute • Demonstrate • Illustrate	• Operate • Perform • Interpret	• Apply • Use • Practice
4. Analysis objectives:	• Solve • Compare • Appraise	• Distinguish • Contrast • Classify	• Differentiate • Categorize • Critique
5. Synthesis objectives:	• Synthesize • Design • Summarize	• Diagnose • Manage • Plan	• Propose • Hypothesize • Formulate
6. Attitudinal objectives:	• Show sensitivity • Respect opinions	• Accept responsibility • Demonstrate commitment	• Be willing to assist
7. Skill objectives:	• Perform • Demonstrate • Show • Conduct	• Compute • Teach • Role play • Take	• Operate • Complete • Design • Do

Some examples of learning objectives that trainers expect participants to achieve are listed below:

Seven Learning Objective Types

Fact objective:
By the end of this training, participants will be able to: List four risk factors for skin cancer.

Understanding objective:
By the end of this training, participants will be able to: Describe three ways parents can protect their children from the harmful effects of UV radiation.

Application objective:
By the end of this training, participants will be able to: Demonstrate their ability to use NCI's Physician Data Query to research information on cancer clinical trials related to two case studies.

Analysis objective:
By the end of this training, participants will be able to: Contrast the barriers to fecal occult blood testing and colonoscopy by naming two barriers that are similar and two barriers that are different.

Synthesis objective:
By the end of this training, participants will be able to: Design an action plan to increase community awareness of the importance of cancer clinical trials through working within their own community-based organizations.

Attitudinal objective:
By the end of this training, participants will be able to: Demonstrate a commitment to increasing the number of women aged 50 years or older who get mammograms by agreeing to tell five friends in the next 3 months to schedule a mammogram.

Skill objective:
By the end of this training, participants will be able to: Perform a correct clinical breast exam using the vertical strip method by demonstrating this to the trainer during a simulation exercise with two standardized patients.

Consider using the "Developing Appropriate Goals and Objectives Worksheet" in appendix B to develop your own training goals and objectives.

2. Selecting Appropriate Training Methods

Suggested Methods for Creating Behavior Changes through Training

To help people gain new awareness and information that will translate into changes in attitudes and behavior, you must choose training methods that correspond to the changes you hope to accomplish. A variety of training strategies will ensure that the learning needs of all types of participants are met. The list below provides some suggested training methods for accomplishing changes in each of these domains. A description of some of the more common training methods, their advantages and disadvantages, and how to implement them follows the list.

Knowledge (Concepts, Facts)
- Computer-assisted instruction
- Discussion
- Field trip or tours
- Films, TV, tapes
- Handouts
- Lecture
- Programmed instruction
- Readings

Attitude (Feelings, Opinions)
- Brainstorming
- Case studies
- Creative arts
- Field trips
- Interview situations
- Open-ended discussions
- Panel presentations of survivors, family members, or health professionals
- Role playing

Behavioral Skills
- Action plans
- Demonstrations
- Guided practice with feedback
- Practicums
- Role playing
- Simulations

Training Methods Overview

The following table summarizes which of the training methods described below can be used to achieve changes in participants' knowledge, attitudes, and behavior skills.

Training Method	Knowledge	Attitude	Behavior Skill
1. Lecture	X		
2. Small Group Discussion	X	X	
3. Brainstorming	X	X	
4. Case Study	X	X	X
5. Demonstration	X		X
6. Role Play	X	X	X
7. Creative Work	X	X	

Note: For tips on how to facilitate an entire training, see Section III.2.

Once you review all of the training methods, consider using the "Training Plan Worksheet" and/or the "Training Plan Template" in appendix B.

Training Method #1: Presentation/Lecture/Panel Discussions

A presentation or lecture can convey information, theories, or principles quickly and easily. Some examples specific to cancer education might be reviewing the epidemiology of a specific type of cancer or reviewing a current screening protocol. Presentations can range from straight lecture to some involvement of the participants through questions and discussion. Presentations depend on the trainer for content more than any other training technique does.

Uses
- Introduces participants to a new subject
- Provides an overview or a synthesis
- Conveys facts or statistics
- Addresses a large group

Advantages
- Covers a lot of material in a short time
- Works with large groups
- Provides context for more practical or hands-on training techniques
- Gives lecturer or presenter more control than in other training situations

Disadvantages
- Emphasizes one-way communication
- Is not experiential in approach
- Requires that participants take passive role in their learning
- Requires that lecturer possess skills as an effective presenter
- Is not appropriate for changing behavior or for learning skills
- Limits participant retention unless it is followed up with a more practical technique

Process

1. Introduce the topic: Tell the participants what you are going to tell them. Use an opening that:
   - Explains the purpose of the presentation and why it is important
   - Relates to the topic, situation, participants, or speaker
   - Involves and stimulates the audience
   - Creates positive thinking and peaks interest
   - Gets attention, for example, by using:
     - Questions
     - Unique facts
     - Illustrations
     - Quotations
     - Brief stories
     - Jokes (in good taste)
     - Gimmicks
     - Compliments
     - Subject matter of significance
   - Serves as a preview to subject matter

2. Present the topic

3. Hold participant attention and interest by:
   - Being enthusiastic, dramatic, or humorous
   - Using specific examples that:
     - Provide clarity, color, and credibility
     - Help a general thought become a specific one
     - Make the impersonal become more personal
   - Avoiding jargon
   - Varying the pace
   - Providing opportunities for participant involvement, by:
     - Questioning both ways
     - Acknowledging individuals, by name, if possible
     - Asking for participant assistance
   - Using references that show material is aimed at a specific group
   - Using surprises and extras
   - Inviting the participants to ask questions

4. Use a closing that:
   - Summarizes the entire activity and emphasizes the key "take home" message
   - Makes a meaningful statement
   - Relates to the topic, situation, participants, or speaker
   - Ties together the activity as an entity

Variations

A lecturette is a term used for a brief (e.g., no more than 15-20 minutes) presentation or lecture. Often these are made more interactive by using a "call and response" format such as interspersing questions to the participants in between lecture points made by the presenter. For example the trainer might ask, *"Which communities or populations are most impacted by cervical cancer?"* After participants offer answers, the trainer could then validate the right answers, correct misinformation or wrong answers, and then briefly summarize the take-home messages. In this manner, participants are acknowledged for what they already know while new and accurate information can be offered by the trainer.

Another variation on the presentation method is a panel discussion. A group of experts (e.g., cancer survivors, family members, or health professionals) present their perspectives to the participants through prepared remarks or spontaneous answers to questions posed by a moderator or facilitator. This approach can be made more interactive by allowing time for participants to ask questions or make comments. A moderator or trainer can model this interaction by asking one or two questions to "prime the pump." Participants can also write their questions on index cards if the size of the training group makes it logistically difficult for participants to ask questions verbally.

Training Method #2: Small Group Discussion

A small group discussion is an activity that allows participants to share their experiences and ideas or to solve a problem. It exposes participants to a variety of perspectives and experiences as they work together to accomplish the task. Some examples specific to cancer education include breaking people into small groups to discuss ways to encourage more people over the age of 50 to have regular colorectal screenings or, for a health care professional audience, ways to improve cancer pain management.

Uses
- Enables participants to present their ideas in a small group
- Enhances problem-solving skills
- Helps participants learn from each other
- Gives participants a greater sense of responsibility in the learning process
- Promotes teamwork
- Clarifies personal values

Advantages
- Allows participants to develop greater control over their learning
- Encourages participants to be less dependent on the trainer
- Encourages shy or less talkative participants to become involved
- Allows for reinforcement and clarification of the lesson through discussion
- Builds group cohesion
- Elicits information from participants

Disadvantages
- Takes time to move people into groups
- Compromises quality control if a trained facilitator is not in each small group

Process

1. Arrange the participants in small groups using some of the ideas listed on page 30

2. Introduce the task that describes what should be discussed in the small group

3. Tell participants how much time they have

4. Ask each small group to designate:
   - A discussion facilitator
   - A recorder
   - A person who will present the group's findings to the larger group

5. Check to make sure that each group understands the task

6. Give groups time to discuss

7. Circulate among the small groups to:
   - Clarify any questions participants may have
   - Make sure that participants are on task
   - Make sure that a few participants are not dominating the discussion

8. Bring all of the small groups together to have a large group discussion

9. Have the people designated by each group present a summary of their group's findings (this could be a solution to a problem, answers to a question, or a summary of the ideas that came out during the discussion)

10. Identify common themes that were apparent in the groups' presentations

11. Ask the participants what they have learned from the exercise

12. Ask them how they might use what they have learned

Determining Group Size

Participants learn through their own experience, especially by discussing questions posed by the trainer. Discussions can take place in a large group, in a small group, or between two participants. The following information is useful in determining the appropriate size of the group for specific activities.

- Most people find it difficult to speak in a group of strangers. Also, there is usually not enough time for everyone to speak. Therefore, if everyone is to participate actively, small groups are essential.
- Most people find it difficult to listen attentively for long periods. Therefore, talks should be short, and people should be given an opportunity to discuss a topic or issue in small groups.
- We all remember much better what we have discovered and said ourselves than what others have told us. Therefore, participants should be given questions leading them to express all they have learned from their own experience first. This needs to be done in small groups.
- A resource person or facilitator can briefly sum up the points from each group and add his or her own insights later, instead of taking a long time to tell people what they know.
- Pairs are useful for:
  - Interviews
  - Intimate sharing
  - Practicing some skills (e.g., listening or feedback)
  - A quick "buzz" with one's neighbor to stir a passion or prompt a sleepy group into action

EXAMPLE For example, if your group consists of breast cancer survivors, participants can pair up to discuss how they felt when they were first diagnosed with breast cancer and strategies they used to cope with their diagnosis.

EXAMPLE If your group consists of health care professionals, they may pair up to discuss how they feel when they have to notify a woman that she has breast cancer and strategies they use to deal with being the bearer of such devastating news.

- Triads (groups of three) are very useful for:
  - Getting everyone to think and participate actively; one can be passive in a group of five, but that is unlikely in a group of three
  - Testing out an idea one is hesitant to present to the full group
- Groups of four, five, or six will add a bit more variety for sharing ideas and insights. Four, five, or six can be a good size for a planning team, a film discussion group, or a more complex situation.

However, the bigger the group becomes, the longer the discussion and the decision-making process.

Dividing Groups and Assigning Roles
When facilitating an interactive training, it sometimes is necessary to divide participants into groups and assign them roles. The following are some imaginative ways to divide participants into groups:
- Deck of cards—the four suits are the four groups
- Colored stickers or dots placed on or under chairs
- Different types of candy (e.g., peppermints, butterscotch, cinnamon, or fruit flavors), which participants pick out of a basket
- M&Ms of different colors
- If groups do not need to be exactly even, use things like types of cars participants drive, types of toothpaste they use, preferences for different types of music, etc.

Selecting a Group Recorder/Reporter
- Select any date at random; the person whose birthday is closest to that date becomes the recorder
- Choose a person who lives closest (or farthest) from the meeting site
- Choose the person newest (or oldest) to the organization
- Choose the person with the most pets (including fish)
- Choose the person who exercises the most
- Choose the person who watched the least TV in the past week

Training Method #3: Brainstorming

Brainstorming is an activity that generates a list of ideas, thoughts, or alternative solutions around a particular theme or topic. Creative thinking is more important during this activity than practical thinking. No idea is dismissed or criticized; anything offered is written down. Often participants stimulate each other's thinking.

After the list of ideas is completed, the group clarifies, categorizes, or discusses one item at a time, depending on the situation. Some examples related to cancer education include brainstorming all the reasons teens start using tobacco or all the barriers to referrals for clinical trial participation on the part of primary care physicians in rural areas.

Uses
- Introduces a problem or question (e.g., *"Let's brainstorm all the reasons women might be reluctant to return for followup after an abnormal pap result."*)
- Forms the basis of discussion
- Can use in conjunction with group discussion

Advantages
- Generates ideas and leads to discussion quickly
- Allows everyone's ideas to be expressed and validated without judgment
- Generates energy to move forward with problem solving
- Stimulates thought and creativity

Disadvantages
- Can be difficult to get participants to follow the rules of not diminishing or criticizing the ideas generated during the actual brainstorming activity
- Affords opportunity for participants to get off track and develop a list too broad to guide discussion
- Opens up the possibility that participants may feel badly if their idea meets with criticism
- Requires that participants have some background related to the topic

Process

1. Establish the rules for brainstorming, including the following:
   - All ideas will be accepted for the list
   - At no time should an idea be discussed or criticized
   - Discussion occurs only after the brainstorming session is complete

2. Warm up the group by doing a "practice" exercise such as having everyone write down on a piece of scrap paper everything you can do with a rule—then go around the room and generate a group list

3. Announce the cancer-related topic, problem, or question

4. Write the ideas and suggestions on a flipchart to prevent repetition and keep participants focused on the topic

Note: It is helpful for your co-trainer to record the ideas while you call forth the ideas from the group. If there is no co-trainer, a trusted participant can function in this role. Be sure, however, that the participant chosen for this recorder role can keep up with a fast-paced generation of ideas. Nothing impedes the brain-storming process more than a recorder who constantly asks for ideas to be repeated, words to be spelled, or acronyms to be explained.

5. Allow silence; give participants time to think

6. Provide positive feedback to encourage more input from participants (i.e., say *"These are great ideas..."*)

7. Review written ideas and suggestions periodically to stimulate additional ideas

8. Conclude brainstorming when no one has any more ideas to add to the list

9. Review the final list before discussion

Variation

A variation to the method described above is to ask each participant to write down his or her thoughts or ideas about the topic on Post-it notes. The trainer then collects all the notes and quickly organizes them into categories. The participant group goes over the categories and responses under each one and discusses the similarities, differences, consistencies, inconsistencies, and take-home messages.

Training Method #4: Case Study

A case study is a written description of a hypothetical situation that is used for analysis and discussion. It is a detailed account of a real or hypothetical occurrence (or series of related events involving a problem) that participants might encounter. It is analyzed and discussed, and participants are often asked to arrive at a plan of action to solve the problem. Case studies can help group members learn to develop various alternative solutions to a problem and may help develop analytical and problem solving skills. Some cancer-related examples are illustrated below.

Uses
- Synthesizes training material
- Provides opportunity to discuss common problems in a typical situation
- Provides a safe opportunity for developing problem solving skills
- Promotes group discussion and group problem solving

Advantages
- Allows participants to relate to the situation
- Involves an element of mystery
- Avoids personal risks by using hypothetical situations
- Involves participants in an active manner

Disadvantages
- Requires a lot of planning time if you need to write case studies yourself
- Requires careful design of discussion questions

Process

1. Introduce the case study to participants

2. Give participants time to familiarize themselves with the case

3. Present questions for discussion or the problem to be solved

4. Emphasize that there is not always only one right solution, if appropriate for the specific case

5. Give participants time to solve the problems individually or in small groups

6. Circulate among the small groups to:
   - Clarify any questions participants may have
   - Make sure that participants are on task
   - Make sure that a few participants are not dominating the discussion

7. Bring everyone back together for a larger group discussion

8. Invite participants to present their solutions or answers

9. Discuss all possible solutions or answers

10. Ask the participants what they have learned from the exercise

11. Ask them how the case might be relevant to their own lives

12. Summarize the points made

Tips for Developing Case Studies

- Develop a case study that is as realistic as possible.
- Describe the people in the case study.
- Use names (but be sure to indicate that they are not the names of real people).
- State their genders, ages, ethnicities, and other relevant characteristics.
- Describe the specific situation.
- Think about the specific issues you want the participants to address.
- Use the case study to challenge assumptions (e.g., health care worker doesn't always know the answers, patients aren't always uninformed).
- Avoid giving solutions to the problems raised in the case study.
- Avoid making the case study too complex or too simplistic.

Some examples of discussion questions that use the adult learning cycle as a model include the following:

- Describe what you see and hear happening in this case study.
- What feelings does the case study evoke in you?
- What are the key issues that are brought to light by this case study?
- What do you think are some of the underlying causes that lead to these issues?
- What are some possible strategies for dealing with these issues?
- How can we each make a difference in addressing these issues?

EXAMPLE

Example Case Study

You have been invited to conduct a training for home health nurses on the topic of cancer pain management. You were told that there are a number of issues that impede the use of appropriate pain medication with cancer patients who are followed by the home health agency. One of these in particular involves nurses not feeling comfortable advocating with physicians for their patients because of fear of addiction to opiate derivatives.

During the training, a nurse participant, Suzanne, brings up a recent article she read in the *New York Times Magazine*. The article described the abuse of oxycontin in rural America. Suzanne says, "There's no way I'm going to contribute to getting a whole generation hooked on those things. I'm just trying to protect my patients' grandkids by keeping those things (oxycontin pills) out of the house." Another participant, Ellen, adds that most of her "little old ladies" are too sensitive to medications to "get them started on something that powerful." You realize that there are a lot of passionate feelings about this topic and wonder how you should handle the situation.

Case study questions for training participants to discuss:
• Describe what you see happening in this case study.
• What feelings does the case study evoke in you?
• How do you think Suzanne is feeling?
• How do you think Ellen is feeling?
• What do you think are the underlying issues behind each of their responses?
• What are some effective ways you, as the trainer, could handle this discussion?
• How will your discussion about this case study influence how you might handle other difficult training discussions in the future?

Training Method #5: Demonstration

A demonstration is a method for showing precisely how a skill, task, or technique should be done. The trainer or a skilled participant shows other participants how to successfully perform a given task by demonstrating it, describing each step, and explaining the reasons for performing it in a particular way. It is often followed by a practice session in which the participants carry out the activity under the supervision of the trainer. The use of models or props (e.g., silicone breast models or fecal occult blood collection kits) greatly enhances a training on self breast exams or colorectal screening. Having simulated or standardized patients for clinicians to practice new skills (e.g., performing clinical breast or pelvic exams) leads to effective acquisition of these new skills.

Uses
- Show participants how to perform a skill (e.g., showing community members how to do a self breast exam or use the collection kit for a fecal occult blood test)
- Clarifies and corrects misconceptions about how to perform a task
- Shows how participants can improve or develop skills
- Models a step-by-step approach (e.g., how to do a clinical breast exam using the vertical strip method)

Advantages
- Provides learning experience based on actual performance and is relevant to the participant's job or personal experience, especially when combined with hands-on practice
- Illustrates processes, ideas, and relationships in a clear and direct manner
- Requires low development costs
- Helps participants' focus their attention
- Involves participants when they try the method themselves

Disadvantages
- Has limited usefulness
- Requires a lot of planning and practice ahead of time
- Requires facilities and seating arrangements that are carefully planned so all members of the audience have an unobstructed view of the demonstration
- Requires enough materials for everyone to try the skill being demonstrated

- Does not ensure that participants will immediately be able to duplicate the skill being demonstrated after seeing it demonstrated
- Requires that participants take passive role during demonstrations which may cause them to lose interest, particularly during afternoon hours and toward the end of the session

Process

1. Introduce the skill being demonstrated: What is the purpose?

2. Present the materials that are going to be used

3. Demonstrate the skill for participants

4. Repeat the demonstration, explaining each step in detail

5. Invite the participants to ask questions

6. Allow participants to practice the skill themselves

7. Circulate around to each person to:
   • Observe participants as they perform the skill
   • Provide them with constructive feedback

8. Bring participants back to the larger group

9. Discuss how easy or difficult it was for them to perform the skill

10. Summarize the take-home messages or key points

Training Method #6: Role Play

Role play is a technique in which several individuals or a small group of participants act out a real-life situation in front of the group. The scenario of the role play is related to the training topic and must have a skill-based objective. For example, in a training on breast cancer for nursing students, two participants might role play how to teach a woman how to do a self breast exam. There is no script; however, the situation is described in as much detail as appropriate. The participants make up their parts as the situation unfolds. The role play is then discussed in relation to the situation or problem under consideration.

Uses
- Helps change people's attitudes
- Enables people to see the consequences of their actions
- Provides examples of possible reactions or behaviors
- Provides a safe environment for exploring problems they may feel uncomfortable discussing in real life
- Enables participants to explore alternative approaches to various situations
- Explores possible solutions to emotion-laden problems

Advantages
- Provides opportunity for stimulating new ideas while having fun
- Engages the group's attention
- Simulates the real world
- Provides a dramatic way of presenting a problem and stimulating a discussion
- Allows participants to assume the personality of another human being—to think and act as another might

Disadvantages
- Requires that participants feel comfortable being in front of a group (some participants may feel self-conscious, shy, or may fear looking "ridiculous")
- Requires dyads or triads in which everyone is either acting or observing to address participant reluctance

Process

1. Prepare the actors so they understand their roles and the situation

2. Set the climate so the observers know what the situation involves

3. Observe the role play

4. Thank the actors and ask them how they feel about the role play (be sure that they get out of their roles and back to their real selves)

5. Share the reactions and observations of the observers

6. Establish ground rules for having a group discussion about the role play. For example:

   EXAMPLE
   - Make your comments in a self-oriented manner. Try to express your feelings as you were watching the role play. For example, *"The interaction in the role play made me feel…"*
   - Make your comments descriptive of what happened. For example, *"I noticed that the woman had eye contact twice with her friend."*
   - Try not to interpret the behavior of the players in terms of why they did what they did. If this seems necessary, however, ask the players in an open-ended way rather than putting words into their mouths (e.g., *"I was wondering why you asked the woman her marital status."*)

As a group leader, your attitude and direction in this discussion are important. Try to protect the role players from too much exposure to negative comments. In addition, try to get the observers to put their comments in the form of suggestions on how to improve the handling of the situation. The best way to do this is to set the example yourself. Attempt to be as nonevaluative as possible. Try to invite people to talk freely about their own experiences. Then summarize the comments given in relation to the learning points.

7. Discuss as a group the different reactions to what happened

8. Ask the participants what they have learned

9. Ask the participants how the situation relates to their own situation

10. Summarize the main messages or points and application

Handling Participant Resistance

There might still be some resistance to role playing. Several types of resistance you might encounter are presented below along with suggestions on handling.

• **Fear of exposure:** This usually relates to a person's fear of being exposed to the total group and acting as a fool. One way of handling this is to use multiple role playing rather than single role playing. Divide the group in pairs and ask them to do their own role plays in different corners of the room. Using this method, you should walk around to get a feel for how each dyad is doing and whether the role play is being used the way it was intended.

• **What is going to happen to me?** Generally this refers to a person's fear of not knowing the procedures involved in role playing. This may be related to lack of knowledge about the topic or lack of role playing skill. Usually a good explanation of the different steps in the session clarifies the issue. You should ensure that people won't be criticized by acknowledging how difficult role plays can be and thanking participants for their bravery in being willing to step outside their comfort zone to provide an excellent learning experience for everyone.

The most important thing in dealing with resistance seems to be to allow it to be there, accepting the feelings and thoughts behind it. But at the same time, you should try to be clear that you want to do the role play and why. If you feel good about it, this will be reflected by the group.

Role Play Example: A Woman with Colon Cancer Considering Clinical Trials

You are Sonya, a woman just diagnosed with colon cancer. You have no medical insurance. You are talking to Mary, the local support group leader, about recommended treatment options. You've heard about clinical trials, but you tell her, "I don't want to be a guinea pig just because I'm poor."

You have heard about the Tuskegee study, in which African American men with syphilis were studied for years without getting treatment. You know that some of your neighbors get paid for participating in asthma studies. You want the best treatment, but you don't want to be treated poorly.

You want to know:
• What are clinical trials?
• Why can't I choose my treatment if I decide to be on a trial?
• What are the pros and cons of participating?
• Are they experimenting on people?
• How do I know I'm being protected?

You are Mary, a local community leader who runs a support group. You want to assist Sonya by helping her understand more about what clinical trials have to offer and refer her to community resources. Talk with her using the following guidelines:
• Be sensitive to Sonya's concerns.
• Remember to provide information that is fact-based, not your opinion.
• Provide resources and support.

During the discussion, you may wish to address the following:
• What clinical trials are
• How patients are protected
• Risks and benefits of participating
• Informed consent
• How to find out about clinical trials in the community that might be appropriate
• Talking about this information with her doctor or nurse
• Talking with her family

EXAMPLE

TRAINER'S GUIDE FOR CANCER EDUCATION

Training Method #7: Creative Work

Although some people believe that using the arts in training is "touchy feely" and therefore not appropriate, others have found that this approach is well received by many audiences. These training activities give participants an opportunity to think or act "outside the box." Examples of creative activities include:

- Making a collage (e.g., make a collage of ways you got support when you were diagnosed with cervical cancer)
- Drawing or painting with markers, water colors, chalk, or colored pencils (e.g., painting a picture of what fear of recurrence looks like)
- Modeling with clay (e.g., making a sculpture of the body post-mastectomy)
- Composing songs, poems, stories, or plays (e.g., writing a play about teens who changed their peer group's norms related to smoking tobacco)

Uses

- Encourages participants to engage the "right brain" (creative, non-linear part), especially important after a "left brain" training method (i.e., didactic or linear presentation)
- Explores other ways to think about familiar situations
- Enables participants to explore emotionally-laden topics in a safe way
- Encourages people to move beyond their comfort zone

Advantages

- Gives participants an opportunity to have fun while dealing with emotionally laden issues
- Allows participants to move around (especially good for kinesthetic participants)
- Provides a creative way of dealing with sensitive issues
- Fosters interaction and emotional connections among participants

Disadvantages

- Requires additional space and materials
- Intimidates participants who feel shy about artistic endeavors (But don't assume that your audience won't respond well to this technique. You might try out the idea with a few people who are demographically matched to your potential participants before your training session.)
- Causes participants who are used to linear thinking and came to the training to get new information to question the usefulness of this approach

Process

1. Introduce the creative activity to participants

2. Discuss how the activity ties into the topics being covered

3. Provide participants the "permission" to take risks, be creative, and not feel that they have to strive for perfection. Sometimes asking people to remember what they were like in the 5th grade will help them to be less inhibited and "let go" of their inner critic

4. Assure participants that these activities are not intended to be judged on artistic merit but rather to stimulate new ways of thinking about the topic

5. Review the materials that are available to complete the creative activity (e.g., clay, markers, magazines, scissors, glue, etc.)

6. Tell participants how long they will have to work on their creations (e.g., minimum of 30 minutes). Explain that you will give them a 10-minute warning before they have to finish their work

7. Provide the allotted time for participants to create

8. Circulate around the room to see how participants are doing

9. Give the 10-minute warning, as promised

10. Bring everyone back together for a larger group discussion

11. Discuss the ground rules for the discussion:
    • Participants should support each other
    • Comments made about another person's creation should relate to how the creation makes them feel
    • Comments should not be evaluative or judgmental

12. Invite individuals to share their creations and how they tie into the topic

13. Ask participants to discuss both of the following:
    - The process of creating
    - The meaning behind their work

    EXAMPLE For example, in a group of breast cancer survivors, each person would share her collage with the group and talk about the images that were selected, the meaning behind them, and how they relate to the support they got when they were diagnosed with breast cancer. Then they would talk about how it felt to create the collage.

14. Summarize the discussion

15. Affirm participant's work and ability to be creative

3. Choosing Audiovisual Materials

Audiovisual materials are essential to effective instruction. The primary purposes of training media are to support the explanations (by illustrating, demonstrating, and emphasizing) and to provide motivation (by increasing sensory appeal, adding variety to the instructional approach, saving time, and retaining participant interest). They can be used to increase knowledge and change attitudes.

Characteristics of Effective Training Media

They should be:
- Simple (easy to understand, uncomplicated)
- Accurate (facts and figures, current information)
- Manageable (easy to operate and manipulate, simple, neat, and practical)
- Colorful (use color to emphasize main points)
- Necessary (illustrate essential materials, contribute to successful accomplishment of learning objectives)

When Selecting Training Media

- Use your training objectives to determine where audiovisual materials are needed to assist participant learning.
- Be selective. Remember that a few good training media will do more for the achievement of objectives than will many confusing ones.
- Update and improve your use of training media or develop new ones for more effective participant learning.
- Consider the enhanced visual/verbal relationship that different media can create. The objective is to maintain visual simplicity and verbal clarity for maximum retention of information.
- Remember that dark rooms can put participants to sleep especially after a meal. Keep the area as well lit as possible while ensuring participants can see the words on the screen.
- Maximize the use of media by following slides, videos, audiotapes, and photos with a targeted discussion. Consider the following format as one useful way to move participants from description, to feelings, insights, and action steps:

- Describe what you see and hear happening in this video.
- What feelings does the video evoke in you?
- What are the key issues that are brought to light by this video?
- What do you think are some of the underlying causes that lead to these issues?
- What are some possible strategies for dealing with these issues?
- How can we each make a difference in addressing these issues?

Main Types of Training Media
- Handouts
- Flipcharts and flipchart paper
- Overhead transparencies and projector
- Computer-generated presentations (e.g., PowerPoint) using computers and LCD projectors or 35 mm slides and projectors
- Videotapes and tape player

Each will be discussed in this section.

Handouts

Handouts are supplementary materials that provide a detailed expansion or reiteration of one or more aspects of the presentation.

Hints:
- Handouts can be your worst distraction during a presentation if distributed while you are speaking. Whenever possible, provide handouts at the end of a presentation unless the audience will use them during the training. In that case, provide the handouts before the presentation to avoid distraction.
- Reduced-size reproductions of charts or slides used during the presentation can be extremely useful to participants as reference material. Adding brief interpretive statements can remind participants of your key points at a later date.

Flipcharts

- A flipchart pad can provide flexibility for developing and modifying simple sketches, diagrams, and statements during the course of a presentation.
- Color is extremely important. Green, blue, and brown should be used primarily for words. Avoid visuals that are one color. Use red, orange, or yellow for highlighting only. If you have five- or six-line visuals, use colors to separate them or to group them.

Hints:
- Maintain the flow of your talk while you write.
- Avoid talking to the board.
- Stay to the side while writing on a flipchart pad.
- Write large and neatly.
- Draw a faint outline of a diagram or model in pencil before the presentation to provide guidelines for the marker or chalk.
- Limit the number of words to avoid pages that are too "busy" and thus distracting.
- If you prefer, have a co-trainer or participant write while you facilitate group discussion.

Overhead Projector

An overhead projector is used to project material from a book or a prepared transparency onto a screen.

Hints for designing transparencies:
- Do not use more than four of five words per line. Keep in mind that the area that can be projected is only 7.5" x 9.5".
- Do not crowd too many lines onto a transparency.
- Design it so it can be read from the back row of the training room.
- Use dark letters on light backgrounds.

Hints for using overhead projectors:
- Place a transparency on the projector before the training in order to focus it.
- Always have a spare light bulb (in case the one provided with the overhead projector burns out) and extension cord with you.
- Designate someone to control the room lights.

Slides, LCD Projectors, and Computers
(for computer-generated presentations)

Slides are still the most common visual aid used in training. However, many health care professionals are switching to LCD projectors and computers to project computerized presentations onto a screen. The following information applies to both slides and PowerPoint presentations.

Hints for designing slides or a computer-generated presentation (e.g., PowerPoint):
• Keep each screen simple with bullet points and simple visuals. Each bullet point can be elaborated during the presentation.
• Use large enough font (30 point) so that the text can be read from the back row of the training room.
• Use colors and designs that are pleasant, but not distracting for the viewer.
• Use colors that make text stand out on a slide. Use a light color for the text on a dark colored background (pale yellow on dark blue is best). The more color used, the less effective it will be.
• Use visual aids that complement the text.
• Use uniform font.
• No more that 75 percent of each slide should have text.
• Use animation (on PowerPoint presentations) sparingly. While it is interesting to have bullet points appear or cross the screen as you read them, too much animation can be distracting.

Hints for using slides:
• Make sure your slides are placed in the carousel so they project right side up.
• Practice showing your slides **before** the training.
• Practice using the remote control for changing slides.
• Practice operating the electronic pointer if you will be using one during your presentation.
• Always have a spare bulb and an extension cord with you.
• Designate someone to control the room lights.

Hints for using an LCD projector and computer:
• If you do not have your own slide projector or LCD and portable computer, reserve one for your training.
• Make sure the computer is equipped with compatible software to run your presentation (e.g., does the computer have PowerPoint?).

- Make sure that your presentation fits onto a diskette, or put it on a Zip Disk. If a Zip Disk is needed, you will need a portable Zip Drive.
- Before the training, do a test run of your presentation to assure that there are no problems using your disk in the computer.
- **ALWAYS BRING A COPY OF YOUR PRESENTATION ON OVERHEADS—JUST IN CASE!**

Examples

Examples of good and bad slides from computer presentations follow:

Bad Example
- Font too small
- Too many words on the slide/screen
- Not visually pleasing

> **Ways to Prevent Skin Cancer**
>
> – Stay out of the sun between 10:00 a.m. and 4:00 p.m. unless you are adequately protected.
> – Wear sunscreen that is 15 SPF or higher. Make sure that the sunscreen has not expired. Reapply sunscreen several times thoughout the day.
> – Be sure to wear long-sleeved shirts, long pants, wide-brimmed hats, and sunglasses.
> – Talk with your friends and family members about sun protection. Remind them to stay away from the midday sun, use sunscreen, and wear full coverage clothing.
> – It is best to combine these strategies to make sure that you are getting full prevention from the sun and decrease your chances of developing skin cancer.

Good Example
- Large enough font (at least 30 point) the slide/screen
- Visually pleasing

> **ABCs of Decreasing Skin Cancer Risk**
>
> **Away**—Stay away from the midday sun
>
> **Block**—Use 15 SPF or higher sun block
>
> **Cover-up**—Wear full coverage clothing
>
> Use a combination of these strategies

Videotape Players

Because the videotape player is extremely versatile, it is rapidly becoming a major tool in presentations.

Hints for using videotape players:
- Use is limited for large groups (i.e., more than 20 participants) because multiple monitors or large video projection screens are needed.
- Most equipment is portable but cumbersome.
- Compatibility of the type and size of the videotape and cassette to the available equipment should be carefully considered.
- Have tapes set at the proper starting point so that only the PLAY button needs to be pushed.

4. Crafting a Realistic and Effective Training Plan

Once you are clear about the characteristics of the participants and the training goals and objectives, you can design a realistic and effective training plan.

It is important to consider not only what you hope to achieve in terms of changes in knowledge, attitudes, and skills, but also the sequence of various training activities and information. There should be a good balance between didactic and interactive activities, between acquiring new knowledge and skills, and having an opportunity to synthesize and apply new information and behaviors. Most trainers design trainings that are too packed with activities and information. While it is important to have additional activities that can be used if needed, it is essential to remember that participants will retain more if given opportunities to reflect, synthesize, and practice new insights and skills. Some guidelines to follow include the following:

Vary Activities
Change the type of activity approximately every 30 minutes (e.g., if you just gave a 20-minute lecturette on a new cervical cancer screening policy, give participants an opportunity to discuss in small groups the implications of this policy on their client base or have participants apply this new information to a prepared case study).

- Intersperse didactic activities such as lecturing and demonstrations with more participatory ones such as small group exercises, individual work, role plays, and a variety of other training strategies.
- Vary learning activities to appeal to all types of participants.
- Structure activities to go from **simple** to **complex** concepts; from **safe** to more **risk-taking** activities.
- Include activities that encourage real-life problem solving.
- Include opportunities for application and practice.

Set Realistic Goals for the Training
- Choose information or skills that participants need to know; not information that would be nice to know.
- Think about your learning objectives (developed in section II.1)

and develop your take-home messages to correspond with them.
- Remember that three to five take-home messages are the most people can retain in a one-day training.
- Match objectives to training and evaluation methods. For example, didactic or lecture methods can lead to knowledge change but probably not attitude change or skill acquisition. Interactive methods can lead to change in knowledge and attitudes. Demonstrations and practice can reinforce skill acquisition.
- Think about how you will evaluate the training.

Be Aware of Time Management Issues
- Build in time for movement from one activity to another. This is especially important if small group breakouts take place in a different room from the main meeting room.
- Build in time for forming small groups.
- Build in some "slush" time to make up for a late start, getting behind schedule because of lengthy discussion, dealing with unforeseen circumstances (e.g., fire drill), or other time challenges.
- Build in time for breaks. Give participants a break no less frequently than every 90 minutes.

Prepare a Clear Training Plan
The level of detail with which a training plan is written depends on a number of factors:
- Is the person who is designing the training plan the same person who will conduct the training?
  - If the training plan is going to be used solely by the person writing it and is a one-time event, then it can be more of an outline with bulleted "talking points" and places to jot down examples.
- Will there be a co-trainer or others who will need to use the training plan?
  - If the training plan is going to be used by more than one person, it needs to be very detailed and explicit.
  - Is the training a one-time event or will it be offered a number of times? If the training will be offered on an on-going basis, it may be helpful to have more detailed notes to avoid "re-creating" the details each time the training is conducted.

Whether you or another person will be conducting the training, it is extremely important that all directions for activities be explicitly written as well as examples of questions to be used to process or discuss the activities. The suggested time allotment for each activity should also be clearly stated as well as the materials needed to conduct all the activities. This level of detail will ultimately make your life easier and will ensure a smoother training program.

A "Sample Training Plan Template" and a "Training Plan Worksheet" are located in appendix B. A sample training plan follows on the next few pages. For this sample,

The left column contains:
- Plenty of blank space so you can jot down your own notes
- A list of training materials that are needed for each portion of the training
- An estimate of how much time it will take to complete each portion of the training

The right column contains:
- Detailed instructions for what to do and say
- Description of how to use any training materials that are needed for each portion of the training
- Lists of possible answers to questions posed to participants during the training session
- Text in *italics* indicates things for the trainer to say to participants

Sample Training Plan

Time and materials	Task	Trainer instructions
60 minutes	Set up room and familiarize self with location	❑ Arrive early to set up the room. ❑ Make sure there are enough chairs and that they are arranged in a circle (around a table) to facilitate participation and discussion. ❑ Organize handouts, training materials, and visuals (e.g., breast models, mammography films). ❑ Locate lights. ❑ Set up and test audiovisual equipment. ❑ Put out refreshments, candies, etc. ❑ Put out a sign-in sheet and name tags. ❑ Make the room more comfortable and enjoyable (tablecloths, decorations, music, etc.). ❑ Locate restrooms, telephones, and water fountains.
10 minutes ❑ Sign-in sheet ❑ Drinks and refreshments	Participant arrival and sign-in	**As participants arrive:** ❑ Ask participants to write their names on <u>sign-in sheet</u>. ❑ Ask participants to write their names on a name tag. ❑ Offer drinks and light refreshments. ❑ Welcome participants and thank them for taking time to participate in this training. ❑ Reassure them that we are going to have fun while we learn about breast cancer early detection measures. ❑ Review "housekeeping" details such as the location of restrooms, telephones, and water fountains.

Time and materials	Task	Trainer instructions

5 minutes
 	
❑ Prepared flipchart – *Agenda*
 	
❑ Prepared flipchart – *Goal and objectives of training*
	Welcome and introduction	❑ Welcome and make brief introductions.
		❑ <u>Refer to flipchart with agenda</u>. Explain that we have a lot to cover, but hopefully it will be interesting and engaging.
		❑ <u>Refer to flipchart with goal and objectives of the training</u>. Explain that the goal of this training is to:
		  • Increase understanding about the importance of breast cancer early detection
		❑ Explain that the objectives of this training. By the end of this training participants will be able to:
		  • Demonstrate steps involved with making an appointment for a mammogram
		  • List at least three barriers women may face to obtaining a mammogram and suggestions on how these barriers can be addressed by health care organizations.
		  • Describe American Cancer Society recommendations for mammography screening.
		  • Demonstrate commitment to increasing awareness about the need for mammography screening by telling at least four friends to schedule a mammogram in the next month.

15 minutes	Icebreaker	❑ Explain that we will be doing a lot of work together today so it's important to know a little about each other.
		❑ Give instructions for the ice-breaker:
		  • In a roundtable format, ask participants to say their name, what they know about why they were given their name (e.g., named after great aunt), or what it means (e.g., the name Athena is the Greek word for "light").
		  • Ask the women if they think their name fits their personality.

Time and materials	Task	Trainer instructions
5 minutes ❑ Prepared flipchart – *Norms*	**Group discussion and group norms** (this will be covered in more detail in section III. 1.)	❑ Explain to participants that setting "norms" or ground rules for the training will help make the training a safe, respectful, and comfortable environment for everyone to learn and share. ❑ Refer to flipchart with norms listed on it. Review each norm and give a brief explanation. • *I'd like to share with you some norms other groups have found useful.* ❑ Ask if anyone has additional ground rules to add. ❑ Post the ground rules on the wall to serve as a visual reminder.
15 minutes ❑ Blank flipchart paper ❑ Colored markers	**Group brainstorm: barriers women may face to obtaining a mammogram**	❑ Explain to participants that studies have shown that many women face several barriers to obtaining a mammogram. ❑ Ask the participants to brainstorm a list of barriers women may face. ❑ Review the rules of brainstorming with participants. That is, that during the actual brainstorming of ideas, nobody should criticize any ideas that others suggest. Ideas will be discussed only after the brainstorming session is completed. ❑ Using a blank flipchart paper, write down the barriers participants suggest.

Time and materials	Task	Trainer instructions
15 minutes ❏ Blank flipchart paper ❏ Colored markers	**Group brainstorm: barriers women may face to obtaining a mammogram (continued)**	Some examples of barriers women may face include: • Lack of insurance to cover mammogram • Lack of transportation to the appointment • Lack of childcare during the appointment • Difficulty in taking time off work for appointment • Embarrassed to disrobe in front of the provider • Fear that the mammogram will hurt • Fear of finding breast cancer • Fear that having a mammogram means that the woman has no faith in God ❏ When the participants are finished brainstorming the list of barriers, add the barriers that may have been missed. ❏ Read through the list out loud, getting rid of duplicate answers or grouping similar types of barriers suggested. ❏ Explain that in the next portion of the training, participants will work in small groups to discuss ways that health care organizations can address these barriers so that more women will be able to obtain mammography screening.

III. Implement

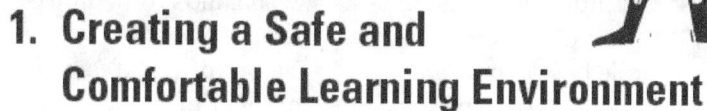

1. Creating a Safe and Comfortable Learning Environment

Adults learn best when the training environment is emotionally safe and physically comfortable. There are a number of different strategies trainers can employ in order to create a positive learning environment.

Setting Up: Ensuring a Comfortable Room Ambiance

Adults learn best in a pleasant environment where their physical needs are met. If possible, when selecting a room make sure there are adequate measures for controlling the temperature. Rooms that have windows that provide natural lighting and contact with the outside world are preferable.

Beware of the following conditions that may distract from the training session:
- Windows that provide outside noise or visual distractions such as people walking by or nature scenes
- Inadequate facilities (uncomfortable chairs, no tables to write on, inadequate lighting, and poor acoustics). Note: For large groups a microphone may be needed. A lavaliere microphone will allow the trainer to move freely around the room.

Sometimes it is difficult to control room conditions. Simply acknowledge to the participants that you are sorry for the discomfort and state what you can and cannot control.

Enhancing the Room

Even the drabbest meeting room can be made more pleasing through the use of decorations. Bring in posters that pertain to your topic, wall hangings, flowers, tablecloths, and candles. Use colorful markers when writing flipcharts.

Setting Up the Room with Chairs

How the room is set up will greatly affect participant interaction. Four common room arrangements and their benefits and drawbacks are described below.

Room Set-up	Benefits	Drawbacks
Circle Seating	• Stimulates interaction • Promotes more equal role between trainer and group members	• Visual aids difficult to use • More difficult if large number of participants • No room to write; materials must be balanced on laps
"U" – Shape Seating	• Leader more easily becomes a part of group • Facilitates communication	• Participants at extremes may be distant from each other—may hamper communication • Takes time to arrange furniture
Workshop Clusters	• Good freedom for participants • Good discussion and diverse communication • Lots of participant working space • Can accommodate large groups	• Takes lots of space • Visuals can be difficult to see
Standard Classroom Seating	• Easy to set up/rented facilities often set up this way • Can accommodate large groups	• Participants cannot easily talk with or see one another • Leader clearly apart from the group • Visuals may be difficult to see

X = Trainer   X = Participants

Getting Started

Once the training room is set up, you are ready to welcome participants to the training. As participants enter the training room, welcome them, ask them to sign in, give them name tags and any training materials or handouts for note taking, and remind them of the starting time. Start the training as close to the scheduled time as possible to signal respect for participants' time.

Help Participants Know What to Expect

Emotional safety is essential in creating a positive learning environment. For participants to feel comfortable in a new training situation they need to know what to expect from the training and what is expected of them as participants. The trainer should review the following with participants:
- The goals and objectives of the training
- An overview of the agenda including:
  - Stop and start times
  - Times for breaks and meals (if appropriate)
- The trainer's role (i.e., a facilitator rather than a speaker or presenter)
- The participants' roles (i.e., active contributors to the group discussions and activities). The trainer should emphasize that the participants have a lot of wisdom to share with the group and that everyone will be greatly enriched if people participate fully in the training activities
- Where they can take care of their basic needs [e.g., location of restrooms, telephones, and places to obtain food and drink (if not provided by the training)]

Learn About Participants' Strengths and Needs

See page 12 for conducting a needs assessment at the beginning of a training if not done before.

Create Ground Rules

Ground rules (also called group norms) are guidelines that help create a safe environment and enable tasks to be accomplished efficiently. Examples of ground rules include:
- Honor everyone's input regardless of educational degrees, professional or community status, or personal experiences with the topic
- Value each person's unique opinions and perspectives
- Agree to disagree, but do so respectfully
- Speak one-at-a-time

- Allow each person time to talk
- Start and end on time; come back from breaks promptly
- Keep personal comments said during the training confidential
- Support those who may have anxiety talking about emotionally difficult topics
- Step outside your comfort zone
- Speak for yourself, not other people (i.e., use "I" statements rather than "everybody" or "other people")
- Take charge of your own learning (i.e., take breaks when you feel necessary, ask for clarification)
- Have fun even though the topic is a serious one
- Ask questions
- Feel free to "pass" when discussing a certain topic

It is preferable for a training group to develop their own ground rules that reflect what is important for them to feel safe. However, if there is limited time, the trainer can suggest a set of ground rules and then ask the group for any additional ones. For example, in professional audiences it may be important to add the ground rule *put all cell phones and pagers on vibrate or turn them off.* The trainer should address any participant concerns about the ground rules and then ask for people to follow these throughout the training. Tape the list of ground rules on the wall so all participants can see them. Refer to them if necessary during the training.

Create a "Parking Lot"

Explain to participants that the parking lot is a place to put questions, comments, or concerns that are important but slightly off the topic currently being discussed. Assure them that everything placed in the parking lot will be addressed by the end of the training (and keep your word, revisiting the parking lot as appropriate throughout the training).

After the trainer has "set the stage" for how the group will move through the training together, she or he can then move into the icebreaker or warm-up activities. Section III.3. describes these in more detail.

2. Facilitating the Training Experience

As a trainer, your goal is to help participants learn new information and build skills. The best way to help people learn is to use facilitation techniques that recognize and build on the knowledge, skills, and experiences they already have.

All of the training methods that were discussed in section II. 2. will be greatly enhanced through the use of good facilitation skills. For some of you, the following information is undoubtedly a review. However, even the most experienced trainers may find a few new ideas or strategies to add to their trainer's tool kit. This section is divided into three parts. The first part covers general guidelines of facilitation and the second part describes effective strategies for working with multicultural training groups. The third part addresses additional considerations.

Part 1. General Guidelines for Facilitation

Encouraging Group Participation

When participants take an active role in their learning, they are more likely to "own" the information and skills covered in the training. People are more likely to participate actively in the training session if you do the following:

- Maintain relaxed body language.
- Use an icebreaker to help participants relax, get to know each other, and get ready to learn. (Specific examples of some icebreakers are described in appendix A)
- Set group norms (sometimes called ground rules) to help make the training a safe, comfortable, and productive learning environment.
- Ask participants to give examples to illustrate a point. This strategy ensures that examples are relevant to participants.
- Bounce back to the group questions you receive from participants, as appropriate. *"What do other people think about this?"* and *"What other ideas do you have?"* are ways to show participants that you recognize their expertise.
- Show participants that you appreciate their contributions by saying things such as, *"That's a good point,"* *"Thank you for bringing that up,"* or *"Many people have that same question."*
- Link discussion back to comments participants made earlier in the session (e.g., *"As Monique (or we) said earlier, this is a very emotionally charged subject."*)
- Bridge forward to what comes next (e.g., *"After break we're going to practice putting these new insights into action!"*)
- Move around. If you stand behind a podium, you are likely to appear distant or inaccessible to participants.

Open-ended Questions

Whenever possible, ask questions instead of talking "at" participants. You can do this by asking open-ended questions—questions that cannot be answered with a simple "yes" or "no." These questions usually begin with words like "where," "when," "what," and "how." The word "why" can be used if it is said in a questioning way rather than a confrontational way. For example, asking, *"Why do you think some people are reluctant to get a colonoscopy?"* would be appropriate, but asking, *"Why aren't you getting regular screenings?"* might be seen as confrontational.

EXAMPLE

Open-ended questions can be used early in a training to get a sense of participants' expectations and baseline knowledge levels. Open-ended questions send the message that participants' input is welcome.

You also can use open-ended questions to review information already covered. For example, you could have participants review or summarize parts of the training by asking the following questions:

- "What new information have you learned?"
- "How will you apply what you have learned today to your personal health behaviors?"

In addition, you can use open-ended questions to help participants share ideas, experiences, barriers, and solutions when you process activities or discuss content. Examples of these types of questions include the following:

- "What has been your experience in finding information about cancer clinical trials?"
- "What are some of the barriers you may face in encouraging your mothers to get mammograms?"
- "How can you overcome the barriers you have identified?"

Open-ended questions are a simple way for trainers to acknowledge that participants have valuable information and experience to share. However, using open-ended questions often takes longer than lecturing. If you find that you are running out of time in a session, you may need to limit responses from participants (e.g., *We have time for one or two more comments.*).

Active Listening

Active listening skills can help participants feel like their ideas are truly an important part of the training experience. In addition, active listening helps the trainers understand participants' concerns. This greater understanding helps you tailor the training to better meet their needs. An effective, active listener uses both verbal and nonverbal skills to acknowledge participation, clarify information, and encourage dialog.

Verbal active listening skills include:
- Repeating what participants say to emphasize their points
- Rephrasing participants' words to see if you understand what they are saying
- Connecting participants' points to something covered earlier in the training
- Asking for clarification if you are not sure what participants mean
- Thanking participants for their contribution

Nonverbal active listening skills include:
- Maintaining open, receptive body language
- Making eye contact with the speaker
- Leaning forward
- Nodding when appropriate

Managing Time

Time management can be one of the most challenging aspects of conducting a training session. It takes a skilled trainer to cover content in a way that involves and engages participants within a limited timeframe. Some ways to manage time effectively are:
- Make clear that participants and trainers will be expected to respect starting, ending, and break times.
- Help participants who wander off the topic to tie in their comments with the discussion at hand.
- Ask participants' permission to "table" questions, suggestions, or comments.
- Limit comments on any given topic. (Always encourage participants to continue their dialog on breaks or after the training session.)

If you run into a situation in which you have too little time to cover all topics on the agenda, you may need to negotiate with participants about what they most want to cover. By allowing them to identify what is most useful to them, you make the most of the time remaining and meet participants' needs.

Giving Feedback

As noted above, it is important to give positive feedback to participants throughout the training. In addition, it may be necessary to give corrective feedback at several points in the training, as you help participants build their skills and knowledge.

TRAINER'S GUIDE FOR CANCER EDUCATION

Effective corrective feedback, which is always given in a supportive manner helps participants improve. Tips for giving corrective feedback include the following:

- Focus your comments on the participant's <u>behavior</u> rather than on the individual.
- Always point out something the participant did well.
- Point out something <u>specific</u> the participant could improve on.

Corrective feedback is never a personal attack on an individual; it is always offered as a way of helping someone increase knowledge or improve skills.

"Checking In" with Participants

A good trainer is able to read the body language of the participants to ascertain the appropriateness of the training content, the pace of the training, and the energy level in the group. This can be done informally on an individual basis during breaks or more formally with the entire group. Asking questions such as *"How's everyone doing?"* (and allowing time for honest responses) or asking people to summarize the key points from a particular segment of the training will help trainers assess whether participants are grasping new information. Mid-training adjustments may need to be made if it appears that many of the participants have not understood the material, appear bored, or need additional help with concepts or skills.

Trainer observations during role plays, demonstrations, or small group activities can provide assessments of how well new material is understood and integrated. For example, if after teaching a group of women how to do a self breast exam, you notice that people are performing it incorrectly during a practice session, you can review and reinforce the correct method. Be careful not to put all of your focus on the one or two "challenging participant(s)" to gauge how the entire group is responding to the training (discussed in detail below).

Working with Challenging Participants

In most training groups there are a couple of participants who pose some challenges to a smooth and effective training process. The table below summarizes some of these challenges.

Types of challenging participants	Why are they challenging?	Ways to work effectively with this type of participant
"Know it alls"	• May actually have a lot of information about the topic but still could benefit from the experiences and perspectives of others	• Acknowledge that they are a wealth of information. • Approach them during a break and ask for their assistance in answering a specific question. At the same time, express your concern that you want to encourage everyone to participate and enlist his or her help in doing so.
"I'm *only* here because I have to be"	• May have been required to attend the workshop, yet has no particular personal interest in the topic	• Acknowledge that you know that some of the participants are present because they have to be. • Ask for their assistance in making this a meaningful experience. • Ask specifically "How can I make this workshop helpful to you?"
"Nay Sayers"	• May be prejudiced • Won't accept your or other participant's point of view	• Don't put them down or make them feel isolated. Keep them involved, if possible. • Throw their views to the group by questions or examples. Try to get the group to bring them around. • Say that time is short and you would be glad to discuss their issues with them individually. • Ask them to accept the views of the group or the trainer for the moment.

Types of challenging participants	Why are they challenging?	Ways to work effectively with this type of participant
"Talkers"	• May be "eager beavers" or show-offs • May be exceptionally well informed and anxious to show it, or just naturally wordy • May need to be "heard" because they are still working through difficult emotional issues • May take time away from other participants	• Don't be embarrassing or sarcastic; you may need their help later. • Slow them down with some difficult questions or difficult tasks (such as group leader). • Interrupt tactfully with something like: *"That's an interesting point… now let's see what the rest of the group thinks of it."* • In general, let the group take care of them as much as possible. • Avoid eye contact. • Give them a role. • State that your role is to keep people on time. • Quick interruption—move to them and put your hand on his or her shoulder. • Paraphrase what they say and move on. • Acknowledge that their stories are important and you and others would love to hear them later or after the workshop.
"Questioners"	• May be genuinely curious • May be "testing" you by putting you on the spot • May have an opinion but not confident enough to express it	• Acknowledge that they seem to have a lot of questions about a particular topic. • If the questions seem like legitimate attempts to gain content information (which other members of the group already know), tell them that you will be happy to work with them later to fill in the gaps or put the question on the parking lot. • Reframe or refocus. Send the questions back to the questioner. • Establish a buddy system (i.e., ask for volunteers who would be willing to meet with them).

Types of challenging participants	Why are they challenging?	Ways to work effectively with this type of participant
"Arguers"	• Have combative personalities • May not want to be at the workshop • May be upset by personal/family health issues • May upset other participants	• Keep your own temper firmly in check. Don't let the group get excited either. • Honestly try to find merit in one of their points (or get the group to do it) then move on to something else. *"That was a good point"* or *"We've heard a lot from [person's name], who else has some ideas?"* • If facts are misstated, ask the group for their thoughts; let them turn it down. • As a last resort, talk with them in private, find out what's going on, and ask for cooperation. For example: say, *"Let's talk at break/end of session. How can we be on the same team?"* • Give them a role.

Part 2. Strategies for Working Effectively with Multicultural Training Groups
Ensuring Cultural Sensitivity

To be effective, trainers must be aware of cultural issues that can affect the training environment. Culture can influence people's values, attitudes, beliefs, and behavior, and therefore has an impact on how people learn, communicate, make decisions, and interact in groups.

Many people think of culture simply as a person's race or ethnicity. However, culture includes many different aspects of people's lives. That is, people's cultural background may be influenced by their:
• Race/ethnicity
• Gender
• Regional differences
• Language
• Sexual orientation
• Level of formal education
• Profession or job
• Spiritual beliefs and practices
• Physical ability
• Age

When you work with multicultural groups, keep in mind that although people from a specific cultural group may share common traits, all members of a cultural group are not alike. Individuals within cultural groups have their own personal experiences, personality traits, values, and belief systems. It is therefore important to respond to a person's needs and not assume that the person will respond in a certain way because she or he belongs to a particular cultural group.

For those of you who train health professionals, keep in mind that there is a "culture of medicine." People who work in health care have a common language and view of health and illness. These views may or may not be shared by community and patient groups. Therefore, when training audiences that are made up of both health professionals and others who do not work in health care, make sure that acronyms, medical jargon, or other abstract concepts are not used unless they are well explained. Also, it will be important to be alert for biases and assumptions that health professionals may share but which may conflict with community members' cultural values, attitudes, and beliefs.

Considering Power Differentials

In training groups where participants might come from diverse backgrounds or positions of power, be alert for ways that power imbalances might affect the training. For example, if you are training a group of health professionals, some may be supervisors of others in the room. The "supervisee" might feel awkward about sharing certain feelings or revealing a lack of skill or knowledge related to the topic with his or her supervisor in the room. Likewise, patients may feel awkward discussing health care concerns if their nurse, physician, or social worker is in the same audience.

Some tips for dealing with power differentials within an audience are the following:
• Acknowledge that the situation exists.
• Emphasize that each person's unique perspective and experience is equally valued and refer to other ground rules that address issues such as these.
• Avoid participant introductions that emphasize academic degrees or professional status. Instead ask people to describe their connection to the topic.
• Lay advocates might need to pair with a health care professional "buddy" when addressing professional audiences so that they can learn what the expected protocol for training these groups is (e.g., Do the professionals want a personal story or a PowerPoint presentation?).

Self-awareness

To fully appreciate cultural power and differences, trainers must:
• Recognize their own culture's influence on how they think and act.
• Understand the complexities of cross-cultural interactions and fully appreciate, value, and respect participants' diversity.
• Be aware of the impact of institutional and societal racism, sexism, ageism, and other such "-isms," and acknowledge how these forms of oppression can influence group dynamics.
• Share appropriate personal experiences from one's "own" culture while not attempting to be an expert on other cultural groups.
• Be aware of their own power within the group and use that power appropriately (i.e., acknowledge that everyone in the

EXAMPLE

room has something important to share and that you, as the trainer, hope to learn from the group).

Cross-cultural Communication

To improve cross-cultural communication skills, trainers should:

- Avoid statements based on stereotypes. If generalizations are used, they should be clearly labeled as such and modified with terms such as "many" or "some."
- Appreciate the different ways that people from various cultures engage in group discussions. Silence, for example, has a different meaning, depending on personal experience and cultural background.
- Ensure that all participants have an opportunity to express their ideas to the group during discussions.
- Remember that participants have different levels of proficiency in reading, writing, speaking, and understanding the language used in a training session.

Finally, even with all cultural considerations in mind, there is no substitute for exercising good common sense and judgment in considering how, what, and when to address various issues in a training. Almost any training activity has the potential to be culturally offensive when facilitated by someone who does not demonstrate respect for participants. Demonstrating respect for participants is crucial and opens the door for mutual growth and learning.

Body Language and Movements

Trainers also must be aware of the different ways people share information. In addition to talking, people use body language, physical contact, and body movements to express themselves. Be aware that the appropriateness of physical space, touching, physical contact, and eye contact can vary depending on cultural norms, personal experiences, and personal preferences.

Part 3. Other Considerations

Other considerations on training facilitation:

- Training team composition sends a message. Whenever possible, trainers' cultural backgrounds should be representative of participants' backgrounds. Diverse groups of participants will benefit from seeing people from their own communities among the trainers. In addition, a multicultural training team models cooperation and sharing among cultures.
- Trainer styles differ, just as learning styles do; therefore, be careful in designing the training on the basis of an individual trainer's preferred style.
- Acknowledge areas of weakness and expertise. If given a direct question, make an attempt to answer it in an accurate and forthright manner. If you do not know the answer, admit it. If you can get back to the questioner with the correct answer at a later date, do so.
- Keep training goals and objectives in mind at all times, but especially when processing. Be aware of participants who might take over or seek to control. If you are uncomfortable with conflict, or uncertain about how to address it, seek training in conflict resolution. Conflict inevitably occurs whenever two or more people come together, so be prepared.

Review the Characteristics of Effective Trainers

Those who are conducting cancer education training programs need to posses certain skills to be effective. Consider using the "Trainer Skills Checklist" located in appendix B to assess your owns strengths and needs.

3. Using Icebreakers and Energizers

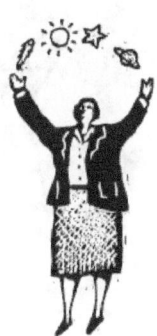

In addition to the training methods discussed in section II.2, icebreakers and energizers are important parts of participatory trainings.

Icebreakers

Icebreakers can be a good way to start your training. They warm-up participants, put them at ease, get people involved, and open up communication. Icebreakers create a positive learning climate within the group. They foster interaction, build group identity, stimulate creative thinking, acquaint participants with each other, and help establish comfort.

Considerations for selecting an icebreaker:
• Think about the group with whom you are working.
• Consider participants' ages, cultural backgrounds, educational levels, occupations, and personalities.
• The length of the icebreaker depends on the length of the training. More time can be devoted to icebreakers when the training is a full day or longer.
• Icebreakers should make people feel comfortable. Do not use an icebreaker which would embarrass someone, or at which people would fail. Use an icebreaker that makes you feel comfortable, not one that raises anxiety.
• Choose icebreakers that encourage everyone to speak. This is especially important for shy or timid participants. Once their voice is "in the room," shy participants are more likely to contribute to subsequent discussions.
• Icebreakers are best when they are related to the topic of the training. However, sometimes it is important to have a "fun" icebreaker not related to the topic to lighten the mood or create a comfortable environment!

Examples of icebreakers are found in appendix A of this trainer's guide.

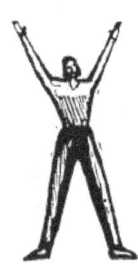

Energizers

Energizers can be used at anytime during a training when the energy or attention of the participants is low. Energizers should take no more than 5-10 minutes. They are really intended to get people up and moving—not to spend a long time discussing ideas. They are especially helpful right after a meal when people are often sluggish.

Introduce energizers with enthusiasm since some participants may be reluctant to "act silly." Model the activity first and be an active participant yourself. This gives participants "permission" to get involved, too.

Examples of energizers are found in appendix A.

4. Conducting Closing Activities

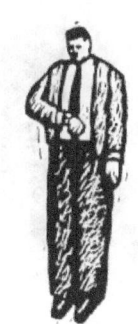

Close the Training

It is important to close a training. Often this step is overlooked due to time constraints. In addition, some trainers feel that the evaluation serves as the closing activity. However, closings are different from conducting an evaluation of the program. They provide a way to summarize or "wrap-up" the training content as well as an opportunity to "close out" the emotional aspects. Done well, they help participants draw a boundary between the training and the rest of their lives and prepare them for the reentry process.

Put Closure on the Content of the Training

Participants should experience a sense of closure with regard to the content of the training. Some examples of ways to do this are listed below:

- Ask for a volunteer to summarize the key take-home messages.
- Conduct games that review concepts or information learned during the training.
- Do a post-test.
- Develop an action plan describing how the participant will use the new knowledge, attitudes, or skills.
- Review expectations from the beginning of the training and ask if all have been met. Answer any lingering questions or concerns.

Trainings where there has been a lot of personal sharing or where participants have formed strong emotional bonds need closure so that participants are not left with unfinished feelings.

Put Closure on the Emotional Component of the Training

Examples of ways to put some closure on the emotions that were generated by the training include the following:

- Take a group photo.
- Have participants stand in a circle and say one thing they have appreciated about the other participants. A variation is to have people write comments on small pieces of paper and put their contributions in cups marked with each participant's name. This strategy works best when participants have been together over a

2- to 3-day training or part of a group that meets over several months.

- Give participants an opportunity to plan a reunion or another time to get back together (again, this is most appropriate for groups that have met over time or where deep bonding has occurred).
- Give certificates of participation or completion.
- Give gifts or incentives as a way to thank people for their time.

An example of a closing statement is located in appendix A.

5. Evaluating the Training

It is important to give participants an opportunity to give feedback about the content of the training, the trainer(s), and the logistics of the training. There are a number of ways trainings can be evaluated—some more formal and some less formal. Ideally the evaluation should relate back to the training goals and objectives. Choose an evaluation strategy that will be most appropriate for your audience. While health care professionals might be familiar with Likert type scales, diverse community groups might prefer a less structured approach. The sample evaluations that follow range from a more structured, quantitative approach to a very informal, qualitative instrument.

Many trainers feel that it is important to wait at least some amount of time before looking at training evaluations. Right after a training you may feel somewhat vulnerable so try to wait until the next day, at the earliest, to review the evaluations. When reading the evaluations, remember that feedback is a gift. Most gifts come from well-intentioned people but not all of them are "on target." Read each evaluation carefully, then review them for themes. Trainers learn most from the reactions of the majority of the participants rather than focusing on one or two comments. Although "outlier" comments can be helpful, most often they say more about the participants than about the trainer or training. If you are using a quantitative or Likert scale evaluation form, enter them into a database if you have one and then review the average scores for each item. If you are using a qualitative evaluation tool, summarize participant comments and reactions.

Finally, in order for evaluations to be most useful, trainers need to develop an action plan for incorporating useful feedback into future trainings.

Examples of training evaluations can be found in appendix A.

IV. Summary and Conclusion

Comparison of Training Elements for Three Audiences

For each training you conduct, you will need to plan Assessment, Goals/Objectives, Training Strategies, Use of Training Media, Icebreakers, Energizers, Evaluation, and a Closing Activity. The chart below summarizes much of the information contained in this guide, and how it applies to running trainings for different audiences.

	Patients/Survivors	General Community *(People not already involved in cancer as a patient or family member)*	Health Professionals
Assessment	• Focus group • Phone or in-person interviews	• Focus group • In-person interviews (e.g., intercept interviews at malls)	• E-mail survey • Fax-back survey • Phone or in-person interviews with key people
Objectives	All seven types may be appropriate according to training goals		
Training Strategies	• Role plays • Small group discussions • Creative strategies • Case studies • Demonstrations • Lecturettes	• Role plays • Small group discussions • Creative strategies • Case studies • Demonstrations • Lecturettes	• Lectures • Case study • Demonstrations • Small group discussions Note: Role plays and other creative endeavors might be appropriate for certain topics
Use of Training Media	• Flipchart • Overhead • Video	• Flipchart • Overhead • Video	• PowerPoint • Slides • Video

IV. Summary and Conclusion

	Patients/Survivors	General Community (People not already involved in cancer as a patient or family member)	Health Professionals
Icebreakers	• Exercises that encourage sharing	• Exercises that introduce the workshop topic	• Brief introductions • Focused on topic of workshop
Energizers	• Fun	• Fun	• Focused on stretching, but not activities that may be perceived as "silly"
Evaluation	• Qualitative tools • Quantitative and qualitative combined for lower-literacy tools may be appropriate	• Qualitative tools • Quantitative and qualitative combined for lower-literacy tools may be appropriate	• Likert, quantitative tools • Qualitative tools
Closing Activity	• What I appreciate about others • What I learned • What I'll do differently as a result of this workshop	• What I appreciate about others • What I learned	• Action plan

Reference List

Armstrong, T. (1993). *7 kinds of smart: Identifying and developing your many intelligences.* USA: Plume.

Arnold, R., Burke, B., James, C., Martin, D., & Thomas, B. (1991). *Educating for a change.* Toronto: Doris Marshall Institute for Education and Action Between the Line.

Centre for Development and Population Activities. (1994). *Training trainers for development.* Washington, DC: Author.

Center for Substance Abuse Prevention (CSAP). (1994). *Facilitation skills development process. Training manual.* Rockville, MD: Center for Substance Abuse Prevention, Substance Abuse and Mental Health Services Administration, Department of Health and Human Services.

De Mauro, D., & Patierno, C. (1990). *Communication strategies for HIV/AIDS and sexuality: A workshop for mental health and health professionals.* New York: Sex Information and Education Council of the United States.

Gesell, Izzy. (1997). *Playing along: 37 learning activities borrowed from improvisational theater.* Duluth, MN: Whole Person Associates.

Hope, A., & Timmel, S. (1995). *Training for transformation: A handbook for community workers* (Rev. ed.). (Vols. 1-3). Zimbabwe: Mambo Press.

Knowles, M. (1990). *The adult learner: A neglected species* (4th ed.). Houston, TX: Gulf Publishing Company.

Kolb, D.A. (1984). *Experiential learning: Experience as the source of learning and development.* Englewood Cliffs, NJ: Prentice-Hall, Inc.

Kroenhart: G. (1995). *Basic training for trainers: A handbook for new trainers* (2nd ed.). Sydney: McGraw-Hill Book Company.

Margulies, N. (1991). *Mapping inner space: Learning and teaching mind mapping.* Tucson, AZ: Zephyr Press.

Markova, D. (1996). *The open mind: Exploring the 6 patterns of natural intelligence.* Berkeley, CA: Conari Press.

Mountain-Plains Regional AIDS Education and Training Center. (1994). *HIV/AIDS Curriculum*, 5th Edition. Denver, CO: Author.

Newstrom, J.W., & Scannell, E.E (1980). *Games trainers play.* USA: McGraw-Hill, Inc.

Newstrom, J.W. & Scannell, E.E. (1994). *Even more games trainers play.* USA: McGraw-Hill, Inc.

Pike, R. (1994). *Creative training techniques handbook: Tips, tactics, and how-to's for delivering effective training* (2nd ed.). Minneapolis: Lakewood Books.

Schott, C., & Phillippo, J. (Eds.). *Expressing our creative selves: A recreational manual for youth care workers.* Athens, GA: Southeastern Network of Youth & Family Services.

Silberman, M. *Active training: A handbook of techniques, designs, case examples, and tips.* New York: Lexington Books.

Swift, R. (ed.) (1998). *The HeART of training: A manual of approaches to teaching about AIDS.* Cooperative Agreements Training Working Group, Special Projects of National Significance Program, HIV/AIDS Bureau, HRSA.

Vella, J. (1998). *Learning to teach: training of trainers for community development.* Washington, DC: Save the Children/OEF International.

Vella, J. (1994) *Learning to listen learning to teach: The power of dialogue in educating adults.* San Francisco: Jossey-Bass Publishers.

Vella, J. (1994) *Training through dialogue: Promoting effective learning and change with adults.* San Francisco: Jossey-Bass Publishers.

Werner, D., & Bower, B. (1982). *Helping health workers learn: A book of methods, aids, and ideas for instructors at the village level.* Palo Alto, CA: The Hesperian Foundation.

Example #1

Icebreaker — Paired Interviews

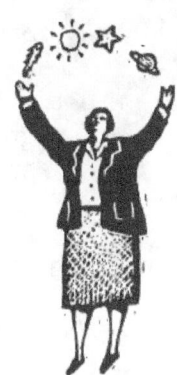

Purpose

To help participants get acquainted with their fellow participants and practice their interview skills

Time

Depends on number of participants. Allow 1 to 2 minutes per participant

Group Size

No more than 20 for one large group; can divide large groups into smaller ones but then everyone would not hear all the introductions

Materials

Scrap paper and pens/pencils for participants to jot down notes

Directions

1. Pass out postcards or playing cards that are cut in half.
2. Instruct participants to find the person who has the other half of their card. (This gets people up and moving around.)
3. When all pairs have matched up, ask them to take turns interviewing each other. Each person will have four minutes to learn the following things about his or her partner:
   • Name
   • How they spend their day (e.g., job or other responsibility like caretaking for a sick spouse)
   • Their interest in or connection to the training topic
   • One hope for the training
   • One interesting thing about them (e.g., hobbies)
4. Tell participants that they will be introducing their partner to the entire group when it reconvenes, so they may want to take notes.
5. After 4 minutes, give participants a signal to change partners.
6. At end of 8 minutes (or after each person has had a chance to be an interviewer and be interviewed), call large group back together.

Appendix A

7. Start the introductions by modeling a succinct introduction of her/his co-trainer.
8. If some participants give lengthy introductions, remind the group that time is limited and it is important to hear from everyone.
9. Assure participants that they will have other opportunities at breaks and meals to network.
10. Thank participants for their introductions.

Example #2

Icebreaker — Go-Rounds

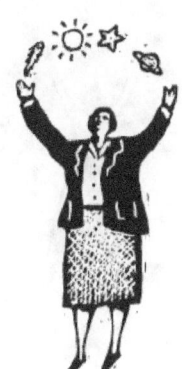

Purpose

To give participants a chance to learn something about their fellow participants and to encourage everyone to speak out

Time

One minute per person

Group Size

No more than 20 for one large group; can divide into small groups but then everyone would not hear all the introductions

Materials

None

Directions

1. State the purpose of the exercise and ask each person to say his or her name followed by the answer to one of the following questions:
   * What is one thing you'd do if you were given $100,000 with no strings attached?
   * What is one thing you'd like to change about the world (or about cancer care, education, or screening)?
   * Describe a strong feeling you've had in the past week and a reason for that feeling.
   * What is one thing you'd like to get from the training?
2. Post the questions on a flipchart paper or overhead so participants can focus on the discussion and not on remembering the question.

Example #1

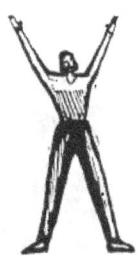

Energizer — Beach Ball Toss

Purpose
To review material learned from a previous session or determine what participants would like during the current session

Time
5-10 minutes

Group Size
No more than 20–25 participants

Materials
Choice of using either a beach ball, Nerf ball, or Koosh ball

Directions
1. Instruct participants to form a circle.
2. Explain that you will throw the ball to someone within the circle. When that person catches the ball, he or she should mention a key message or concept heard during a previous session.* Once he or she has made a statement, he or she should toss the ball to another person within the circle.
3. Ask participants not to toss the ball to the person on their immediate left or right.
4. Suggest that participants should step out of the circle once they have participated.
5. Continue tossing the ball until all participants have had an opportunity to participate.

*Note: If this is the first session for the training program, ask person to tell you what he or she expects to learn.

Example #2

Energizer — That's Me

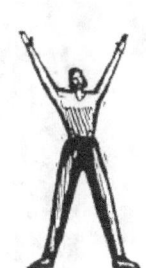

Purpose

To get participants moving, i.e., standing up and down; it also allows participants to get acquainted with each other

Time

5-10 minutes

Group Size

Unlimited

Materials

None

Directions

1. Give the following directions:
- You will ask a question, such as "Who has grandchildren?"
- If that characteristic "fits," participants will stand up, raise both arms outstretched over their head, and shout,
  "That's Me!"
2. Ask the group to practice standing up and shouting
   "That's Me!" when you count to three.
3. Ask the group as many of the following questions (or questions of your choice) as time allows. Mix in questions that are more personal with those that pertain to the topic of the training.
- Who lives in (this state)?
- Who traveled more than 4 hours to get here?
- Who has grandchildren?
- Who exercised this morning?
- Who took a vacation last summer?
- Who ate at least one serving of fruit this morning?
- Who had a clinical breast exam within the last year?
- Who watched at least one movie or videotape in the last month?
- Who plans to shop while in (this city)?
- Who knows someone who has been on a cancer clinical trial?
- Who has a pet?
- Who has read a nonfiction book in the last 3 months?
- Who is eager to learn more about (the topic)?

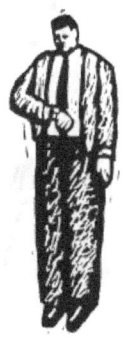

Closing Activities — Closing Statements and Handout

Some activities serve to close out both the emotional aspect and content of the training. This exercise is an example of one that serves both purposes.

Purpose
To give every participant a chance to summarize their experience of the training in a way that the group can share

Time
10-15 minutes

Group Size
Up to 20 participants

Materials
Closing statement handout for each participant

Directions
Ask participants to:
1. Take a Closing Statements Handout (see below).
2. Take a minute to complete any of the sentences on the handout that they choose (give participants 5-10 minutes to complete handout).
3. Form a circle in (the back of the room).
4. Ask participants to go around the circle and share one of the closing statements out loud.

Notes to Facilitator
- You can place this before or after the evaluation, but don't hurry it. Give people a sense of how much longer you plan to keep them (i.e., *"We'll do this exercise for 10 minutes, spend 5 minutes finishing evaluation forms, and then we'll adjourn"*).
- Be sure participants will be able to see and hear each other.
- Don't respond to what is shared; model respectful, quiet acceptance of what's offered.
- End by thanking everyone for sharing the training with you.

Closing Statements Handout

Please complete any of these sentences to summarize your experience of this training event. You will be asked to share one with the group.

I learned…_____
_____
_____

I feel…_____
_____
_____

I was surprised…_____
_____
_____

I'm wondering…_____
_____
_____

I've re-discovered…_____
_____
_____

I figured out…_____
_____
_____

I appreciated…_____
_____
_____

I felt challenged…_____
_____
_____

I'm clearer about…_____
_____
_____

Example #1

Training Evaluations — Form (Version A)

Name (Optional) _____

Were the overall program goals met? _____
_____
_____

Goal 1: The overall goal/purpose of the training is to provide health
education coordinators with the knowledge and skills to plan,
implement, and evaluate effective outreach strategies for
increasing the number of adults aged 50 years and older who get
colorectal screening at appropriate intervals.

❏ Yes   ❏ No

Goal 2: A second goal is to provide health education coordinators with
the knowledge and skills to provide tips for training peers to
conduct effective outreach for colorectal screening.

❏ Yes   ❏ No

If no, please explain and give suggestions for improvement:

1. What are the top three things you learned from this training? _____
_____
_____

2. If you could give the trainers one piece of advice on how to improve the
training, what would it be? _____
_____
_____

3. What were some of the training's highlights or parts that you valued most? _____
_____
_____

4. What did you like least about the training? _____
_____
_____

5. What other types of training would you like? _____
_____
_____

6. What problems or dissatisfaction did you have with the way the program was scheduled? _____
_____
_____

Example #2

Training Evaluations — Form (Version B)

Circle the appropriate response.

1. Trainer organized the material effectively.

Strongly Agree   Agree   Neutral/   Disagree   Strongly
                                       No Opinion   Disagree

Comments:

2. Trainer managed discussions effectively.

Strongly Agree   Agree   Neutral/   Disagree   Strongly
                                       No Opinion   Disagree

Comments:

3. Trainer used effective teaching methods.

Strongly Agree   Agree   Neutral/   Disagree   Strongly
                                       No Opinion   Disagree

Comments:

4. Trainer used handouts and audiovisuals that were appropriate and contributed to the presentation.

Strongly Agree   Agree   Neutral/   Disagree   Strongly
                                       No Opinion   Disagree

Comments:

5. Discussion materials were clear.

Strongly Agree   Agree   Neutral/   Disagree   Strongly
                                   No Opinion   Disagree

Comments:

6. The training can be applied to my current job.

Strongly Agree   Agree   Neutral/   Disagree   Strongly
                                   No Opinion   Disagree

Comments:

7. The material presented is useful on a personal level.

Strongly Agree   Agree   Neutral/   Disagree   Strongly
                                   No Opinion   Disagree

Comments:

8. The material presented is useful on a professional level.

Strongly Agree   Agree   Neutral/   Disagree   Strongly
                                   No Opinion   Disagree

Comments:

9. Would you be interested in attending a followup session on this topic?
  ❏ Yes   ❏ No

If yes, specify the areas that you would like to see included in the agenda.

Example #3

Training Evaluations — Feedback Cards Exercise

Purpose
To provide a mechanism for participants to give feedback regarding the training/learning experience

Time
5-10 minutes

Group Size
Any size

Materials
Two colors of 3" x 5" index cards, enough for each participant to receive one card of each color

Directions
1. Pass around two stacks of 3" x 5" index cards. Each stack should be a different color (best to use colors that are easily distinguishable from each other, e.g., blue and yellow).
2. Ask each participant to take one card of each color.
3. Ask each participant to write, *"One thing you really liked or appreciated about this training (or this day of training) on the ____ color card."*
4. Ask participants to write, *"One thing you wished had been different about this training (or this day of training) on the ___ (other than in step #3) color card."*
5. When all participants have completed the cards, ask that they pass both cards to the front.
6. Thank participants for their input and assure participants that the trainers will carefully consider their feedback.

Example #4

Training Evaluations —
Head, Heart, and Feet Exercise

Purpose
To evaluate the session at its conclusion, especially useful for audiences with limited literacy skills

Time
15 minutes

Group Size
Any size

Materials
Evaluation sheet for each participant, flipchart, markers, and tape

Directions
1. Hand out the evaluation sheet that follows. Explain its objective and how the information will be used.
2. Invite participants to use the markers to draw their head, heart, and feet on the paper.
3. Ask participants to fill in the form (individually or with someone else).
4. If there is time, ask them to share something they learned or to give final comments.

Variation
Draw a large head, heart, and feet on flipchart paper and post it. Distribute small slips of paper and ask participants to write down the major things they learned or got out of the event. Post these points in the appropriate position on the flipchart and discuss them.

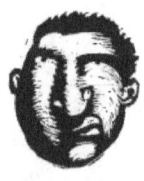 Head: What did you *learn* today?

 Heart: How did today's training *feel* to you?

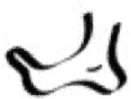 Feet: What are you going to *do* as a result of the training today?

Example #5

Training Evaluations — Faces Exercise

Please circle the face that best describes your feelings about each given training activity:

Icebreaker

Lecturette on risk factors

Values clarification exercise

Small group exercise on barriers and facilitators

Video

Energizer

Role play exercise

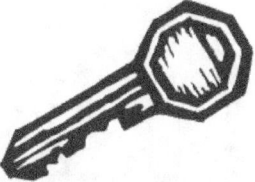

Trainer Skills Checklist

Think about your own skills as a trainer then read through the following statements.

- **Put a check** beside all of the statements you feel describe your strengths.
- **Circle the box** beside the statements that describe areas where you'd like to improve. Think about one or two things you could do to build on your strengths to address areas that need improvement.

☐ You know yourself. You are confident and fully prepared. You are just nervous enough to keep alert.

☐ You know your subject matter. You have studied your topic and have experienced the events about which you speak.

☐ You know your audience. You respect and listen to the participants. You call them by name, if possible.

☐ You are neutral and non-judgmental. You validate everyone's experience and their right to individual perspectives. You respect differences of opinion and lifestyle.

☐ You are culturally sensitive. You are aware that your own views and beliefs are shaped by your cultural background just as your participants' cultures shapes their perspectives.

☐ You are self-aware. You recognize your own biases and "hot-buttons" and act in a professional manner when your "hot-buttons" are pushed.

☐ You are inclusive. You encourage all participants to share their experiences and contribute to the group learning process.

☐ You are lively, enthusiastic, and original. You use humor, contrasts, metaphors, and suspense. You keep your listeners interested and challenge their thinking.

☐ You use a variety of vocal qualities. You vary your pitch, speaking rate, and volume. You avoid monotones.

☐ You use your body well. Your body posture, gestures, and facial expressions are natural and meaningful, reinforcing your subject matter.

☐ You make your remarks clear and easy to remember. You present one idea at a time and show relationships between ideas. You summarize when necessary.

Appendix B

❏ You enhance with illustrations. You use examples, charts, visuals, and audio aids to illustrate your subject matter.

❏ You understand group dynamics, and the stages all groups go through. You are comfortable with conflict resolution.

❏ You are flexible. You read and interpret your participants' responses— verbal and nonverbal—and adapt your plans to meet their needs. You are in charge without being overly controlling.

❏ You are open to new ideas and perspectives. You are aware that you don't know all the answers. You recognize that you can learn from participants as well as offer them new knowledge or perspectives.

❏ You are compassionate. You understand that much of the material may have an emotional impact on the participants. You are empathetic and understanding about participants' emotional reactions.

❏ You are interested in evaluating your work. You encourage co-trainers and participants to give feedback.

Describe one or two steps you can take to improve your skills as a trainer:

_____

_____

_____

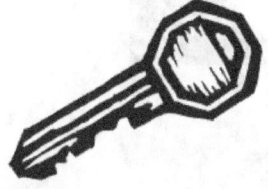

Training Assessment Worksheet

This worksheet will help you conduct a needs assessment for each training you are planning.

• What information do you need in order to design an effective training? (Logistics, content, format, etc.)

• What do participants already know about the topic?

• What experiences or insights related to the topic do participants already possess?

• What do participants believe are the challenges or barriers related to the issue? (For example, why do they think people do not avail themselves of colorectal screening services?)

• What do participants hope to gain from the training? (This includes new knowledge, skills, resources, etc.)

• What do participants desire regarding the logistics of the training?
  ❑ Location of training
  ❑ Length of program
  ❑ Optimal number of days of training
  ❑ Best day of week
  ❑ Time of day

• Which is the most effective assessment strategy for your audience?
  ❑ E-mail survey
  ❑ Fax-back survey
  ❑ Mail survey
  ❑ Telephone survey
  ❑ In-person interview
  ❑ Focus group
  ❑ Review of previous training evaluations

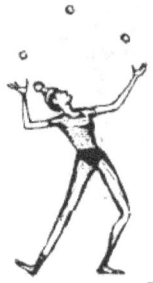

Questions to Help Define Appropriate Training Plan, Goals, and Objectives

This worksheet will help you prepare your plan, goals, and objectives for each training you are planning.

Who are your participants?
• What is their educational level? _____

• What is their experience and skill level? _____

• What gender and age are they? _____

• Are they employed? _____

• What kind of work do they do? _____

• Do they work together? ❑ Yes ❑ No

• What is their literacy level _____

• How many will there be? (approximately) _____

When will you conduct the training?
• What day of the week? _____

• What time of day? _____

• What time of the year? _____

• How long will the session be? _____

• What will be the length of the entire program? _____

• How much time is there for recruitment? _____

Where will you conduct the training?
What is needed?
• What size room is needed? _____

• What equipment is available? _____

• What other supplies are needed? _____

Location
• Is the location accessible? ❑ Yes ❑ No

• Is the location easy to find? ❑ Yes ❑ No

- Can it be reached by public transportation? ❏ Yes ❏ No

- Is there safe parking? ❏ Yes ❏ No

- Is it handicap accessible? ❏ Yes ❏ No

- Is it a place that does not have negative connotations for intended participants? (e.g., some places are associated with poor service or indigent care which may make some participants uncomfortable) ❏ Yes ❏ No

What will the training involve?
- What will be the content of the training plan?

_____

- What training tools will be needed?

_____

_____

- What participant materials and resources will be needed?

_____

_____

- Will there be advance work for participants? ❏ Yes ❏ No

What is the _purpose_ of the training?
- What changes in knowledge, attitudes, behaviors, and skills are you hoping to accomplish through the training?

_____

_____

- What are the goals and objectives of the training?

_____

_____

How **will you do it?**

- How will you enroll people for the training? (Some possible recruitment strategies include flyers, PSAs on TV and radio, ads in newspapers and newsletters, and word of mouth.)

_____

_____

- How will you engage participants?

_____

_____

- How will you get feedback or evaluate the effectiveness of your training?

_____

_____

Sample Training Plan Template

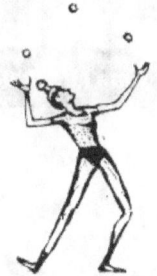

Time and materials	Task	Trainer instructions

Time and materials	Task	Trainer instructions

Training Plan Worksheet

This worksheet will help you plan a training.

Goal:

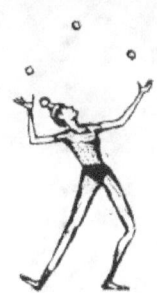

Objectives "At the end of the workshop participants should be able to…"	What content is needed to meet the objectives	What strategies are needed to deliver the content (list 1 strategy) and regulate the energy flow (icebreakers, energizers)	How much time should be allotted each strategy
• List at least 3 barriers women may face in obtaining a Pap test	• Barriers specific to Pap tests on part of the individual woman • Barriers specific to the health care organization	• Brainstorming list of barriers • Reading focus group quotes from women in the community	• 20 minutes • 15 minutes

EXAMPLE

Worksheet for your training:

Developing Appropriate Goals and Objectives Worksheet

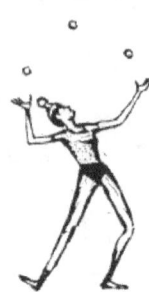

The goal for my training is:_____
_____

The changes I want to see as a result of my training are:
❑ Increase in knowledge:_____
_____
_____

❑ Newly acquired skills:_____
_____
_____

❑ Changed attitudes (e.g., more compassionate, etc.):_____
_____
_____

❑ Increased proficiency in existing skills:_____
_____
_____

Based on the above, the most appropriate objectives for my
training are:
(Please feel free to use verbs located on page 20 for guidance)

❑

❑

❑

Notes

www.ingramcontent.com/pod-product-compliance
Lightning Source LLC
Chambersburg PA
CBHW081501170526
45166CB00008B/2508